Dementia: A Love Story

Readers are encouraged to go to
www.MissionPointPress.com to contact
the author or to find information on how
to buy this book in bulk at a discounted rate.

MISSION POINT PRESS

Published by Mission Point Press
2554 Chandler Rd.
Traverse City, MI 49696
(231) 421-9513
www.MissionPointPress.com

ISBN: 978-1-950659-94-4
Library of Congress Control Number:
2020924734

Printed in the United States of America

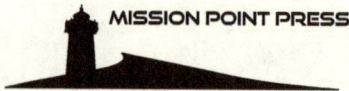

DEMENTIA
A LOVE STORY

by STEPHEN LEWIS

MISSION POINT PRESS

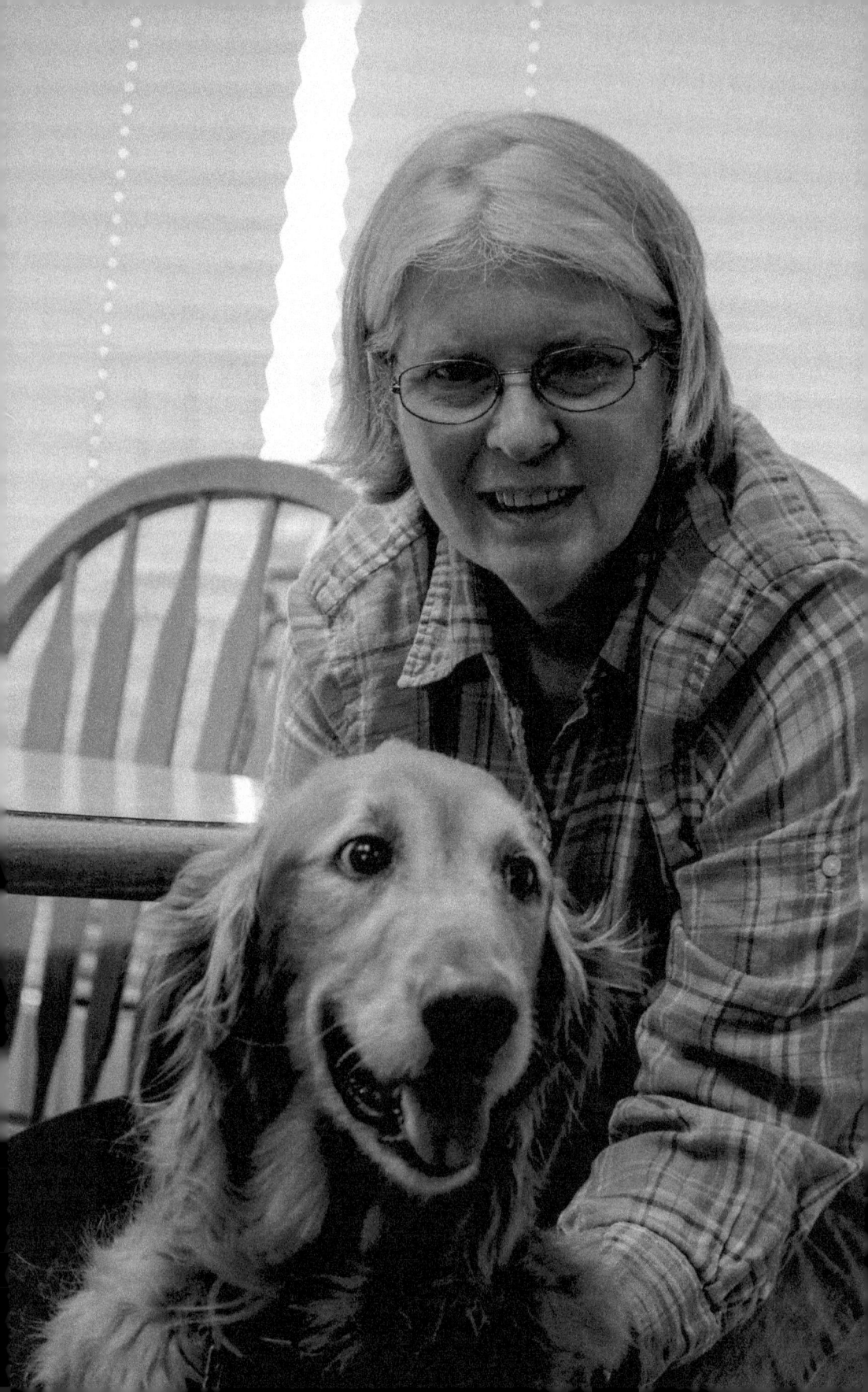

Foreword

I lean over the hospital bed on which lies my wife Carol.

"I'm going downstairs to tread," I say. "Now, you stay right here until I get back. No partying, right?"

Her face breaks into a smile, followed by a laugh.

Other times, when I am holding a fork laden with food in front of her mouth, I have to say her name with sharp emphasis several times to get her attention and redirect her to the task at hand. She starts as though being brought back from someplace else.

At sixty-four, she has early onset dementia, a disease for which there is no cure, only palliative measures.

It wasn't supposed to happen this way. I am ten years older. We didn't talk about her taking care of me into my dotage. We did not have to. Of course, she would. In my mind, I would be Henry Fonda, she Katherine Hepburn on our own Golden Pond. But her disease has turned that actuarial prospect upside down, and it has fallen to me to take care of her. I most willingly undertake that job despite having no preparation for it, as she would have done for me. Our lives together these past thirty-five years, beginning with our improbable meeting—Carol from a farm on hundreds of acres in rural northern Michigan, Steve from a two-family house on a street in Brooklyn, New York—has been a love story in which our divergent backgrounds only strengthened our melding into one indivisible union, and a love story of a different sort it continues to be.

I began writing this journal at the suggestion of a former writing student who thought it might be helpful for me, and that, in effect, I had a responsibility to use my writing skills to produce something that would resonate with others dealing with this disease.

<<< Carol and Abby, not long before dementia hit.

5

That advice worked well for me in several ways. The first had nothing to do with my student's recommendation. It gave me a writing project. I know this about myself, that as long as I am writing on something my world is in order. If I am not, I feel unmoored.

Secondly, to serve the purpose of sharing with other sufferers, I decided to turn my journal entries into blog posts. In doing that, I put myself on a regular posting schedule, which demanded I keep at the task, a kind of deadline pressure that I, in fact, enjoy, having learned to deal with it working on my college newspaper.

I had never written a journal before. As a student of literature, I had dipped into writers' journals, such as those by Hawthorne or Thoreau. I suppose for them, the journals were a kind of storehouse of material that could be mined at a later date for other purposes.

Without any real preconceptions for mine, I just began writing. That is my usual, highly intuitive approach to writing. I start putting words down and see where they will lead me, even in clearly structured writing situations, such as an in-class essay exam, expecting a controlling idea to emerge, which it usually does.

What occurred to me, then, as I began writing this journal, was to start each entry by indicating factual circumstances, such as time of day, weather, physical location of me and Carol, and the dog. Somehow, my mind always needed to locate the dog.

Then, I would respond to whatever prompts my memory might serve up. These prompts often recalled events experienced recently. These events rode along two tracks. One was our continuing day-to-day business, mundane tasks, such as food shopping or other household-related happenings. The other track involved Carol's condition and its treatment by me along with relief aides, therapists, and medical practitioners.

These two tracks were parallel, but they occasionally touched each other when memory created an intersection where something in one track could be illuminated by something in the other. A frequent sort of such intersections would involve a then and now contrast: Carol as she had been versus Carol as she now was.

That contrast creates the emotional core of this book. It is, of course, as it must be, only from my perspective. Other caregivers of dementia sufferers will no doubt recognize the sadness, mixed with anger, at the cruelty of this disease as it ever so slowly, imperturbably, erases the identity of a loved one for both the sufferer and the caregiver.

I have to imagine that process is a constant in all similar cases. But I would argue it is more shattering to observe in early onset cases, such as this one, where it so strikingly affects a person who until its onset was in full control of his or her powers.

With all that in mind, I invite you into this record of our world as we together journeyed to that "undiscover'd country," Hamlet's words for death but an apt descriptor for dementia, a country in either case, from which no traveler returns.

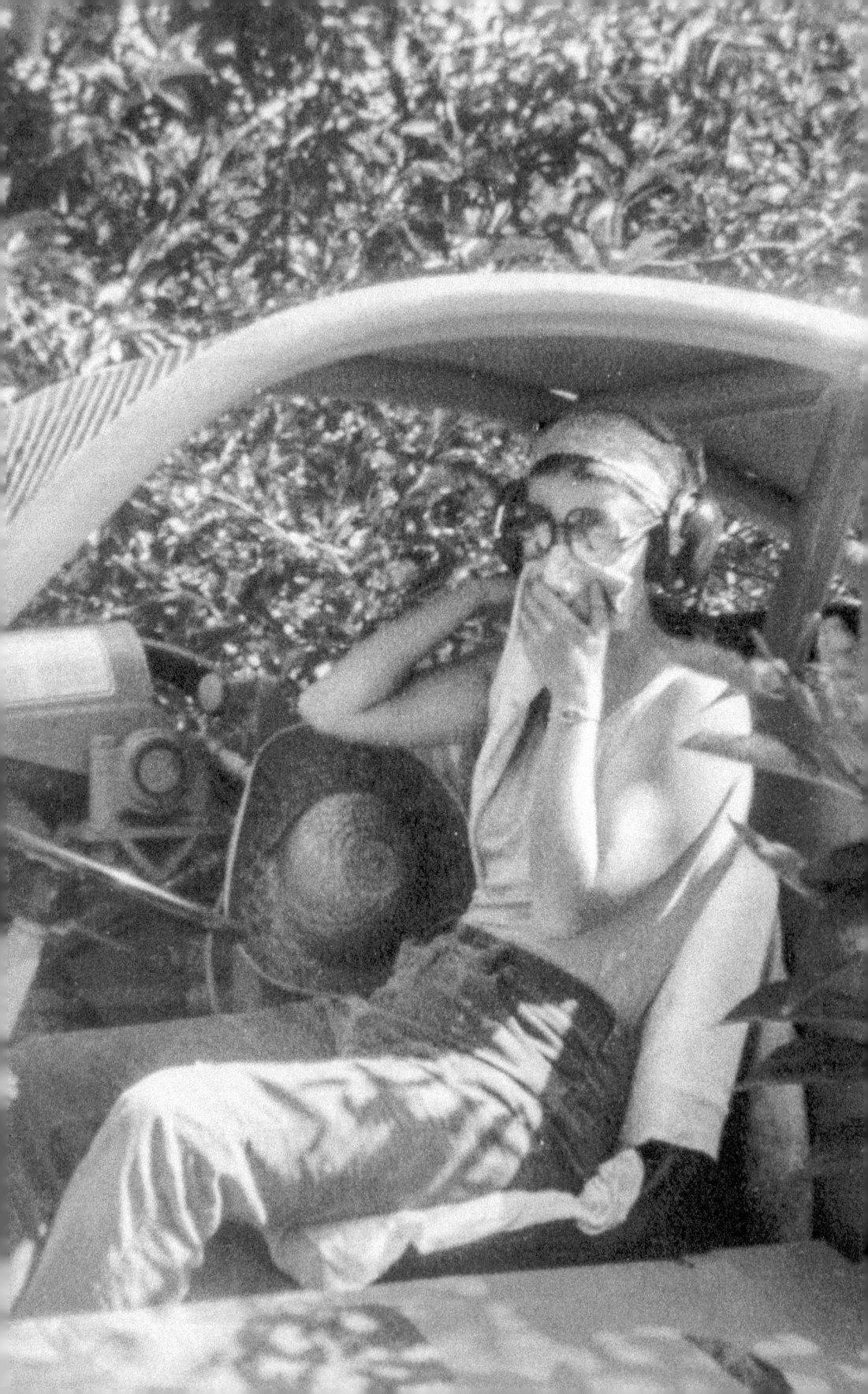

Like Sand Through My Fingers

Sunday night. I just watched an episode of Poldark *on* Masterpiece. *We always watched the PBS shows on Sunday night:* Downton Abbey, *of course, the mysteries,* Sherlock, *whatever was on. We would have after-dinner snacks while we watched, usually hummus and crackers, or sometimes soft pretzels like those sold off carts back in New York, only these are frozen, thawed in the microwave after adding the salt from a packet. But tonight, I watched alone, without a snack, my company the dog who was probably disappointed there were no crumbs to be gathered from the floor.*

Herein is the conflict I wage with myself. The more I fully accept the role of caregiver, the more I must let go of the shreds of our past life together that remain in the occasional smile, or squeeze of her hand in mine, the good morning greetings we exchange during which I tell myself that she knows who I am, the snippet of conversation concerning our daughter now living in Minnesota, all these moments pushing against my exchanging, in totality, my role as husband for that of caregiver.

It is not that I don't want to take care of her, as best I can. Of course, I do. We used to joke that given the fact of my being ten years older, there would come a time when she would push me around in my wheelchair. Her disease has reversed that prognosis, a prognosis that did not include losing my cognitive ability as she has lost hers. The idea was that my body would have weakened, not my mind. In our present here and now, her body is still quite strong as evidenced by the deep bruise she left on my bicep when in a panicked fear of falling she clutched me there.

<<< Carol in the cab of a cherry shaker.

She was always physically strong and capable—the first woman shaker-driver harvesting cherries among the orchards on Old Mission Peninsula, competent behind the wheel of any vehicle, a splendid driver and horsewoman, a serious walker, and even more recently, before her cognitive decline, she was out there shoveling the edges of our driveway missed by my snowblower.

I don't think she has lost much of her strength. What she has lost is both the control of her muscles, and, more importantly, the confidence to use them.

Her continued physical strength contributes to my difficulty in letting go of her pre-disease self and accepting her here and now self, with all its difficulties. Part of me, a persuasive part, insists on trying to retain some sense of normalcy in our daily lives.

That is like clenching my fingers around sand that sifts through my fingers.

It cannot be done.

But the friction of the hard grains against my flesh is its own reward.

I have yielded to some realities. Some time ago, I bought her pants in a smaller size to recognize the weight she has lost, a purchase aided by the advice of my eldest daughter then visiting with her family from New York. Those pants now rest, neatly folded up in our bedroom. I no longer clothe her every day. Given her incontinence and inability to be easily transported to the bathroom, it just makes more sense, as my younger New York daughter suggested when she visited a little time after her sister, to keep Carol in night clothes. So, I bought her two new night garments, appropriate for fall weather, and will add to them a couple suitable for the cold winter approaching.

But, to this point, I have not given in to the suggestion of renting a hospital bed, which would make tending to her easier than her current residence on the living room sofa. I see that advantage, but it is insufficient to overcome the feel of a hospital room that the bed would impose on our living space.

Presently, we both sleep on our L-shaped sectional, and I savor the physical proximity, even though we are not side by side. I hear her breathing, her responding to auditory hallucinations, and sometimes, a frightened call prompted by a sense of falling even when she is lying flat on her back. In the morning, I bend myself around the corner of the L to get near enough to her to hold her hand or stroke her cheek. She sometimes rejects those gestures as an unwanted intrusion of the here and now into wherever her mind has carried her. But, most times, she is accepting, and I feel comforted.

For the most part, our lives follow the same dull routine. In this regard, I am reminded of an observation offered by Thoreau toward the end of *Walden* concerning how easy it is to fall into a repetitive pattern. He notes, to his surprise, how quickly and beneath his conscious notice, his feet produced a path, or perhaps more to the point, a rut between his cabin and the pond, as he traveled back and forth each day for his ablutions.

And so it is with our lives, with very little variation from day to day. But every once in a while, something occurs to me that pushes its way through the dull routine and obliges me to deal with this vexing conflict between the past and the here and now. Such a moment was prompted by my seeing in my email inbox a notice presenting the agenda for the upcoming meeting of the local historical society.

Even before we moved here from New York, Carol's father, a local historian, invited us to come along to a meeting of the historical society. Although I was then still just beginning to learn how to navigate the culture shock caused by introducing my Brooklyn formed self into the wildly different mores of rural northern Michigan, I have always enjoyed learning about history wherever and whenever the opportunity presents itself. Carol savored the chance to share her father's interests and join them to her own.

Once we became residents here, we quite naturally continued attending the society's meetings. We were, in fact, the only members of Carol's extended family who did so, and we continued our participation in the society after Carol's father lost his battle with pancreatic cancer. And then, not for the first time, in another instance of a familiar pattern in my life according to which I, without any obvious ambition, wind up in a position of leadership, I found myself president of the society.

All of which is preamble to the moment when I saw the meeting announcement. I decided I would like to go, mingle again with the folks I had not seen for some time, and just get out of the house for a while and leave my caregiver responsibilities for a couple of hours. None of that gave me any pause. There was, of course, the issue of finding someone to stay with Carol. That, in itself, did not raise my conflict.

What did cause the conflict to raise its troublesome head was what should I tell Carol. Deep into our rut, I never go out in the evening. And I always tell her where I am going, even if it is to walk across the road to our mailbox. She would love to go, I thought, and would be seriously disappointed if she were to stay home while I attended a meeting of the society her father had helped found. She had served as co-editor with me of the organization's newsletter, and had, in short, been more strongly invested in the society than I had been.

I was trapped in the past and unable to see myself in the here and now. My concern about her feelings was based on the woman she used to be. The woman she is now hardly remembers the society, and even if she were upset at my going, as unlikely as that would be, she would in all likelihood not remain unhappy for more than a few minutes as this incident, like all others, simply would not find a foothold in her memory.

When I did tell her where I was going, she offered a glimmer of a smile and nodded.

Unaware, she too, was so deep in the rut she could not see over its top.

Two Steves

Near midnight, after a mixed day, half irritating, half enjoyable. The irritations involved dealing with caregiver relief scheduling difficulties and insurance reimbursement issues. Spent my morning dealing with both. I felt for a while as though I were again the college administrator I once was, sitting at my desk, fielding problems as they arose. I am good at that kind of work, but do not want to do it now. The pleasure was my Tuesday afternoon lunch at neighbors Brad and Amy's house, which provided lively conversation on topics both trivial and important.

Late as it is, I want to work on this piece. I wrote it as a draft some time ago and think here would be a good place to insert it.

The most difficult then versus now tug-of-war in Carol's mind for me is the one where she prefers her memory of me to the actual, present-day me. On more than one occasion, she has consistently demanded to see her husband when I have been sitting right next to her, even holding her hand.

At those moments, I suppose, if she recognizes me at all, I am her caregiver, the guy who attends to her needs. I can insist, as I have done, that the Steve she is remembering is the same Steve talking to her at that moment, but she is not moved. She looks at me as though I have been talking in a foreign language, or if not, have been saying something so palpably false that she need not give my assertion a moment's thought.

What this tells me is that her long-term memory is far more vivid than any present reality. She seems to have, in fact, a tenuous grip on what I've been calling the here and now. Why this is so, is perhaps because her brain simply does not retain much memory of the immediate past, by which I mean the minutes before the present moment. It's as if every moment in the present is a new dawn with no antecedent to provide context.

This might be a bit of an exaggeration, but not much. She does seem to retain memories of things that have bothered or annoyed her. For example, at mealtimes, which she continues to take while still on the couch, I generally get her into something like an upright sitting position. I do this by first swinging her legs over the side of the couch, and then gathering her in my arms and lifting her until she is at least mostly upright. We repeat this procedure three times a day. Apparently it has left something of an impression in her brain, a newly minted memory, for she will react by saying— depending upon her mood—either a simple "okay," or "not again." In either case, she recalls what we are about to do.

But this is the exception. More generally is the rule that a minute or two after any incident, snippet of conversation, or activity, it is as though it never happened.

So, I can understand why she denies that I am who I am, preferring to dwell on her stored memory of who I was.

But understanding it does not make it any easier to deal with, especially when she is in some sort of distress. There was an incident involving the physical and occupational therapists combining to work with her to see if putting a weighted vest on her chest would enable her to resist the rising panic caused by getting on to her feet. In so doing they met significant resistance. She became very angry and fearful at the same time and insisted that she wanted her husband.

That I was standing right in front of her did not satisfy her. I was not the husband she remembered. I was this other guy. On occasion, giving me the small victory of my name, she acknowledges that I am one of the two Steves in her brain.

But she so clearly prefers the other Steve, the one she remembers. I try to close the gap between the two by citing the facts of our lives together: where we met, when and where we married, where our daughter is now living in Minnesota, and so forth. She easily accepts that all of that information is correct, even offers a bit of a smile as her mind fastens on to this or that detail. Nonetheless, she does not connect any of it to me. All of it belongs to that other Steve, and there it will remain.

It is all so understandable.

Caller ID

For now, back into my long-established writing slot of late at night—it is coming on eleven o'clock—when the house is quiet. The dog has settled into her bed, Carol is sleeping, albeit restlessly, on the couch, and I sit across the room with my laptop on my lap.

I usually wake up at this time, my natural biorhythm at work, but tonight will probably be different. Last night, Carol talked from about ten in the evening until four in the morning. I tried several times to calm her down, to ease her into a sleep mode, but with little success. Consequently, I could not fall fully asleep until she did, and then she was up at about eight. I went through the day on four hours of sleep, including a trip to town for groceries.

I have no idea what she was talking about all that time, as her words were not fully nor clearly articulated, and even when I did make out what she was saying, I had no context into which to put it.

Since Carol will turn sixty-five in January, and thus go on to Medicare, we have been bombarded both by postal mail and by calls on our landline with pitches for supplemental coverage. Because my employer-based insurance will provide that supplemental coverage for her, I am not interested.

I toss the paper pitches into the garbage. I deal with the phone calls by paying attention to the caller ID. Some of the callers identify themselves, discernible even through the garbled attempts of the phone to state or display the caller's name. Others come in as just a place name or toll-free number. For those, I pick up the phone and hang it back down again, just to get rid of it without providing an opportunity for a message to be left. On occasions, I will let the answering machine take the call when what shows up on caller ID is a plausible connection, even if I don't recognize it, or if I am awaiting a call that might come in from that place or on a WATS line. Once or twice this process has yielded a conversation with a person I actually do, or should, know.

All of which brings me to why these calls are in my mind today. There were more than the usual number that I permitted the answering machine to take, and so I was reminded to check our outgoing answering machine message to confirm that it was in Carol's voice. I wasn't sure because I had not listened to that message since we installed these phones at least ten years ago.

It turned out that it was her voice, and that raised the question in my mind as to whether under present circumstances I should record a new message. The thought occurred to me that it might be a little strange or awkward for Carol's sister or brothers, or one of our good friends, to hear her voice on the answering machine as though she were still functioning as she had been. I recognize this is unlikely because I am home nearly all the time and I will pick up the phone as soon as the caller ID tells me the caller is someone I know.

I am not sure if others would even have such a thought, but I am sometimes somewhat literal minded, and so it strikes me as perhaps not quite right to have Carol's voice answering our phone when she would not at this point recognize the caller's name.

But besides being occasionally literal minded, I also sense connections that push beyond the first thought. In this case, that is what happened. I am reminded that Carol was determined to have her presence fully established in our relationship. She did not hyphenate her last name, but she usually did keep her maiden name as a middle name. She published her stories as Carolyn Johnson Lewis. That is how her name appears on her driver's license. And where possible, she wanted her name on our various household accounts. Thus, many of the bills we get come to us under her name, and she is listed as the owner of our joint checking and savings accounts.

This never bothered me. In fact, when we were first

together, she handled the bills while I was working several jobs to keep us afloat while dealing with child support payments. Even, in retrospect, I understand that she would have wanted to be the bill-payer anyway. Coming as she did from a culture that even now is traditional in its attitude toward gender roles, she desired to break out of that female subordinate position and establish herself on an equal footing.

She was, in short, insistent about establishing her own identity.

Which is what she is losing, thanks to her disease.

Made even more poignant for me as earlier today, in response to my thinking about our greeting message on the answering machine, I played it. And when I did, I heard her voice, both warm and professional and welcoming.

It hurt a lot.

If I erase that voice on the outgoing message, I will not hear it again.

And I will have taken another step, however grudgingly, away from the then and into the now.

Fear

Afternoon. I am back on my perch in the living room while Carol is on hers, sleeping noisily on the couch. It is a fall day outside, gray and rainy, the leaves on our abundant and ancient maples presenting their speciously bright colors red, orange, and yellow, before dying and falling into brown heaps.

The oak woodwork on the staircase leading to our upstairs communicates a structural strength that is yet insufficient to persuade Carol to climb the stairs to the two landings and through the two turns to reach the hallway leading to our bedroom.

In fact, her condition has worsened beyond her inability to climb steps.

She will not stand though her legs are quite strong enough to support her.

Her fear is stronger still. I can lift her to her feet, but she tries to sit back down, and I wind up supporting all her weight until I can steer her back onto the couch.

Thus, her fear of falling is now crippling, creating in her a paralyzing panic, even sometimes—and this is a crucial point—when she is lying flat on her back. This fear does not seem to result from her memory of a fall. I don't think she now remembers the one she had some ten or twelve years ago, which gave her a broken ankle. No, it seems this fear arises from the lack of communication between her eyes and her brain. I can only try to imagine how disorienting it must be to not know, literally, where my body is, but that is my guess as to what causes her debilitating fear.

Evidence for this hypothesis comes from at least two professional sources. At a routine eye exam about a year and a half ago, she could not read the chart. She could see it, but she could not read it. Her brain did not understand, or perhaps receive, the images from the chart brought to it

Stephen Lewis

through the agency of her eyes. The doctor checked her vision as he would a preliterate child by shining a light through her pupils and declared that her vision was good. Further back, when she had recently finished a course of chemo, I was taking her to an occupational therapist at the local hospital to see if she could recover her beautiful handwriting and the ability to read without losing focus. At that point, her brain was doing a much better, but still inadequate, job of deciphering images presented to it. The therapist noticed that Carol was only comfortable walking down the long, wide corridor leading to the therapist's room when she was next to the wall. Apparently, that proximity to something large and solid enabled her to place her body in relationship to the physical space through which she was moving.

Because of our present living arrangements—sleeping on the sofa in the living room—I do not spend much time upstairs. In the morning, I go up to our bedroom to get fresh clothes and to shower. I visit my office in the room adjoining our bedroom to get used to the new desktop computer I purchased recently when my old one, with all of our financial records, as well as various writing projects, showed signs of its impending collapse. I don't know when I will start working more on it and less on this laptop.

When I do go into our bedroom, I see the new sheets on our bed, which I bought not that long ago, when there was still hope that Carol would be able to overcome her fear and make it up the stairs. I walk past her dresser. On its crowded top are pictures, including a shot of the teenaged me, one of herself and older brother as children, and another of our daughter as a pretty, young girl. Along with the pictures, there are also feathers in a little vase and a small drum, both indicators of her interest in things Native American, and in one corner shoved against the wall, a purse she will never again carry.

In fact, the whole house is permeated by her presence.

Her personality is inescapable; it thrusts itself at you.

She stamped her identity with the artwork depicting scenes of the Great Lakes; with the old violin hung on the living room wall, along with its bow, recalling her love of music; and with the Kodak Autographic Junior on yet another wall bespeaking her love of photography, for she was above all a highly visual person. All over on tabletops and windowsills, her idiosyncratic interests—stones and pieces of wood she picked up on walks, anything that struck a chord in her deeply imaginative mind, triggering memories of her childhood here, her fascination with all things local, lighthouses, evidence of Native Americans' ancient presence, and, perhaps above all, the topography, the bays, the hills and woods, and the farms—for all of it she found a way to place it in our living space.

But there are also the more mundane reminders of the once but no more: the two pairs of winter boots in our bedroom that she will never wear, the watch on her dresser bought on a birthday, worn hardly at all for it soon became clear she could not read the dial, the wonderful winter coat I found online for her on a spectacular sale, the books in her bookcase, anchored on the bottom shelf by her law tomes, the rest reflecting her interests in women's history, women writers, and politics.

All of this is best described as bittersweet.

Sweet because of how these specific items remind me of our shared lives, how dominant she was in shaping our mutual environment.

Bitter because those specifics no longer connect to her mind in any meaningful way.

And how sad that her fear prevents her from moving through and appreciating the environment she created.

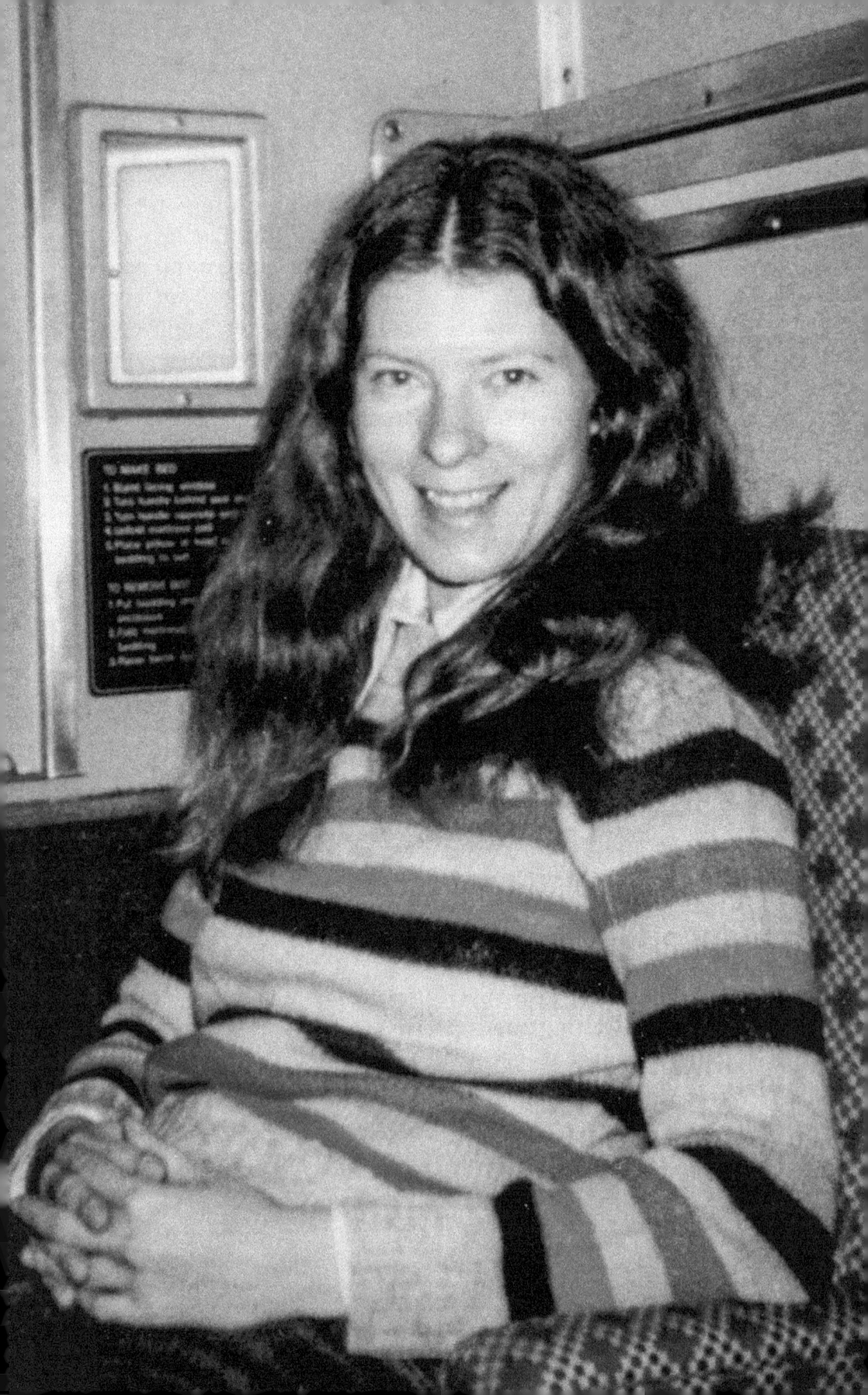

Carol That Was, Carol That Is

Coming on midnight after a long and mostly difficult day, as Carol was in a combative mood. The day was brightened in the afternoon by my walk next door for lunch and conversation hosted by my neighbors Amy and Brad. Amy is dealing with her own medical issues as she has just finished a course of chemotherapy and will be beginning stem cell therapy to deal with myeloma in her spine. She remains her energetic and welcoming self, and along with Brad they have set up these Tuesday occasions for me when I have caregiver relief.

It is becoming increasingly difficult to see in Carol the woman she was, that set of qualities and characteristics being slowly driven out by the insistent presence of the Carol she now is.

I want to fix the Carol that was in my memory to push back against the insistent pressure of the Carol that is.

And will become.

I can do that by cataloging things in our house that predate the onset of the disease.

In our dining room we have the bottom piece of a second-hand breakfront we bought years ago. It had a top section to sit on it, but the only place we could put it was in front of a beautiful old window looking out of the front of the house, so we sold the top piece at a yard sale. I have no idea what the buyers intended to do with it.

The piece we have is about seven feet long and a foot and half deep, providing a large surface, which Carol has filled with all sorts of stuff. There is the antique typewriter in the middle, which amuses and interests the grandkids when they come. Next to the typewriter is a tiny little book of

<<< Carol in her late 20s.

23

bound pages. Most are blank, but on a few in barely discernible pencil strokes are short passages, some seemingly personal, others apparently copied from some source, such as the one suitable for a headstone. I will now never know where this book came from, or who might have written on its pages. Beneath it are two very old volumes. One is Elizabeth Barrett Browning's *Sonnets from the Portuguese*. The second and larger volume is a leather-bound collection of Longfellow's poetry. It was once owned by a Johnson, but I cannot read the first name. Perhaps it says "Mary," which would be Carol's mother.

It makes perfect sense that Carol would have books occupy a place of honor on this piece of furniture. She was—I started to write "she is" and had to correct myself—a book person. She smiled when she told me how her father would find her under a tree reading when she was supposed to be whacking weeds. One of the saddest consequences of her disease is that she can no longer read and has little patience being read to, something which she used to thoroughly enjoy.

Much of the rest of the surface holds photographs, mainly of Carol's family. Prominent among these is an 8×10 picture of Stella, her paternal grandmother, wearing netting over her face as she tended her bees, the necessary agents of fertilization for the family's fruit orchards. Other pictures include one of Carol and Dean, her older brother, as young children. Tucked into the frame of a photo of Carol when she was perhaps in her thirties or early forties standing before the columned front of a public building, maybe in Washington D.C., one of our travel destinations, is the high school picture of one of her best friends. There is a hodgepodge of other pictures: a shot of me and our daughter in England, one of us with the two couples we used to socialize with regularly, a picture of members of the local historical society in front of the Hessler Log House, moved and restored by the historical society. Toward the back-left corner, not visible behind the photos, is a silver tray on top of which is a silver salt and pepper set, somewhat tarnished. These items I am reasonably sure came from her mother, probably passed down from her southern grandmother. Right behind and to the left of the tray is my space in which sits a trophy I received as most valuable player on my sandlot football team, and next to it a picture of me receiving it, with my father by my side. I mention this at this point only because that trophy from more than fifty years ago was buried in a corner of a closet until Carol insisted we take it out, polish it up, and display it. It thus represents the Carol that was in her feelings for me.

On the walls of our downstairs living space are, with one exception, pictures she has chosen, such as the one of the French fur traders in a canoe. Upstairs in her office, her computer has a number of files in which she was laboring to begin a novel for which that print could serve as a cover. Her focus would be on the Native Americans. The French would be there as an excuse for the story to begin. The last story she published a couple of years ago featured a missionary priest, a young Native American woman, and a wolf.

Other pictures include a rendering of the Edmund Fitzgerald going down, and in another frame a startling image of a lighthouse keeper standing atop his building as storming waves rise to his feet, both reminding me of her love of water, and the Great Lakes in particular. She never did fully share my passion for ocean waves and beaches, preferring the calmer grandeur of the lakes.

Also, on this wall, there is a well-executed watercolor of the buildings of Fishtown in Leland on the Leelanau Peninsula, across West Bay from where our house sits on Old Mission Peninsula. She saw the picture hanging in the infusion room where she was getting her chemotherapy, and as was her wont, inquired about it, and found out that the artist was local. Either he, or perhaps his wife, had sat in the same room. We contacted him and bought a print of the picture.

The only non-Carol picture on these walls is an impressionistic image of a jazz musician that hangs above the piano Carol used to play. It is a print from a slide given to me years ago by one of my writing students at Empire State College on Long Island, New York. As I recall, he was an older man, a better artist than writer, but as was usually the case with students at Empire, strongly motivated to succeed.

I pause to look at this catalog from a different angle: those pictures Carol bought to show her connection to my background and interests. In our little TV room, the one we call the green room for the obvious reason of that color on its walls, there is the famous print of a photograph showing workmen calmly sitting high up on a steel beam, part of the skeleton of the rising Rockefeller Center, eating their lunch. One can only wonder where the photographer was.

I began this survey of the artifacts in our house that expressed Carol's interests. Then, I turned to those that she had bought specifically for me. I will conclude by combining these perspectives where our love for each other found its most appropriate place. While Carol was finishing her undergraduate degree at New York University, she moved to an apartment in a brownstone in Brooklyn, my hometown. We enjoyed spending time on an elevated walkway called the Promenade in Brooklyn Heights, which offered a view of Manhattan across the East River. On the wall over the fireplace in the living room is a print she bought representing that place and that view. In my office upstairs is another of Carol's choices for me: the official team photo of the World Series-winning 1955 Brooklyn Dodgers.

Besides pictures, there are the workspaces. To write, Carol demanded isolation. We began by setting her up in the partially finished basement with a desk. When we decided to turn the basement into a little apartment for the convenience of my New York daughters and grandchildren, she lost that space. Nothing else was available in the house. Our daughter still occupied her bedroom, and my office had been, from the beginning, in the remaining bedroom. So, we contracted with our nephew to deconstruct and reconstruct a small outbuilding that the previous owner had used to house a horse. He made it into a rather nice office. I believe it already had electricity, but we had the Internet wire brought out to it and supplied it with a phone line and a walkie-talkie to communicate with me in the house. We furnished it with two desks, one regular flat surface, and one for the computer. Because Carol was heavily into her photography interest at that time, we also put a large cabinet, designed to hold photographic prints. In it now, as well, is the professional grade Canon inkjet printer with which Carol started a business turning her photographs into saleable items.

None of this, however, got much use. Winters made the building difficult to get to. It had no bathroom. In it, however, I recently found a notebook in which she was writing notes to herself in an attempt to get her French fur trader novel into gear. I have only glanced at it, but in the proper mood when I want to bathe in my memories of the writer Carol was, I will sit down and read it.

When our daughter moved out, Carol took her bedroom for her office, and we bought another desk for it, leaving the other office furniture in the little building, which we came to call the barn studio. She worked well in her new in-the-house office, writing her stories and organizing them into a collection we hoped to sell.

Then came her cancer, and subsequent decline. Her office now houses medical assistance equipment, such as the shower bench she no longer uses. Her laptop sits on the desk, next to the phone extension. It's a lovely place to work, looking out as it does at the orchards across Center Road.

A lovely place, but I'll leave it as it is.

It belongs to the Carol that was.

Sackett Street

Late afternoon. It will be dark soon as we crawl toward winter. We've already had two or three light snows, but today the temperature is in the fifties. Back from my Tuesday lunch during which, at my suggestion, we discussed the options available to me as the lease on my Nissan Altima soon expires. I professed my love for the latest gadgets available in the newest models, an argument against deciding to purchase my current lease car. It was pleasant to talk about something, which in any serious way, is not consequential.

The tentacles of the past continue to wrap around me. In truth, I do not fight too hard to free myself from them. To do so would place me in the immediate present facing an inevitable and devastating future. In that respect, reminders from the past, though still painful, serve the useful purpose of turning my mind away from that eventuality.

The reminder that just intruded itself into my consciousness came from a review of a new Thai restaurant. I came upon the review while skimming through the headlines on the online version of the *New York Times*.

I am not particularly a connoisseur of Thai cooking. I believe the last time I had Thai food years ago, I suffered an allergic reaction. The ethnicity of the food did not attract me to the review.

The location of the restaurant did.

It is in Carroll Gardens in Brooklyn.

On Smith Street.

Not far from Sackett Street.

Where Carol rented her apartment while working and finishing her undergraduate degree in the Gallatin program at New York University.

Sackett Street, a short hop from Brooklyn Heights where

we would sometimes dine at a café on Montague Street. We delighted in starting our meal with dessert, usually chocolate mousse, and then a cocktail. After eating, we would walk down Montague Street and onto the Promenade and find a bench. There we could gaze across the East River to the Manhattan skyline, see the World Trade Center towers, and to our north the ancient grandeur of the Brooklyn Bridge. The promenade would usually be busy with joggers, bicyclists, parents pushing strollers, people strolling and talking, or listening to the music in the headphones attached to their Walkmans, that ancient device that played the even more ancient cassette tapes.

Those were hectic times. I was working full time but also teaching overload courses, and adjuncting at Empire State College. Carol was finishing her BA degree and working at the handicapped desk in NYU's library.

In a year or two, she would finish her degree, join me out on Long Island, marry, and together we would buy a house and start our family while she completed her JD at Touro Law Center. She was eight months pregnant when she graduated.

All of that was to come.

But the time on Sackett Street remains prominent in our—I should say my—memory. And in my memory, I recall how fondly Carol spoke of that neighborhood in my hometown of Brooklyn, how she felt comfortable, being looked after by the Italian grandmothers sitting out on their stoops, calling her a good girl and keeping an eye on her as she went to school and came home from work, and how once in her hurry she left her key in the front door and it was still there when she came home. And that memory also brings back to me my connection to the place I had left so many years ago, the whole experience serving as the basis for my poem, "A Street in Brooklyn," celebrating how our backgrounds came together, and I recall how Carol as guest editor of *Dunes Review*, a local journal, published that poem.

In Brooklyn.

On Sackett Street.

So long ago.

A tendril from the past that clutches me in its grip, causing pain at what has been lost but also sending a warm breeze of memory.

A Down Staircase

Just finished my Sunday night television watching, a mix of baseball playoffs and Masterpiece. *Sitting in our TV room I was keenly aware of the empty chair next to mine where Carol would sit on these Sunday evenings, and I was struck by the thought that down the road I might well be rattling around this big old farmhouse by myself.*

For now, in our living/bedroom, she is lying across the room from me on the sofa, talking as she sometimes does, more or less in her sleep, to some voice in her head.

I imagine that one could construct a graph where the horizontal axis would represent time, and the vertical would indicate positive or negative states of mind. For non-dementia people, a positive jump up might occur at that time when some goal was achieved, such as a promotion or finding a romantic partner while a negative step down would occur when a job was lost or a romance ended.

But the ups and downs on such a graph for Carol since the onset of her disease would not involve any of those kinds of life events. Rather, they would correspond to cognitive, emotional, or physical changes as her disease runs its destructive course. There would be few upticks and steady incidents of downward motion from which there would be no recovery. Visually, that horizontal line would move along on an even keel for a while, then drop down, then continue on the lower level, until it dropped again, and so forth, sort of like the elongated image of a staircase.

A down staircase.

Certain objects in our house could be placed on those steps down.

For example, there is the cane in the corner next to the bookcase. It represents the decline in her ability to walk, first noticed at a visit to the lakeside home of our good

friends Marcy and Bob, who had invited us out for a boat
ride. Walking along the plank path leading to the water,
Carol was unsteady. Marcy suggested she might be having
a vision issue related to her glasses. I suspect she was half
right. Eye to brain, but not the glasses. When the unsteadiness continued after fiddling with the glasses, we got the
cane for her without knowing that the dementia had started
to work on her.

As she began using the cane, other accommodations had
also to be made. Her unsteadiness posed a problem in the
bathroom where stepping into the tub shower became difficult. I remembered the grab bar at her mother's house and
installed one on the wall next to the tub, and another, which
used powerful suction cups, on the tiled wall in the shower. .
Even with these aids, she would sometimes grab the towel
rack for additional support, as she stepped out of the tub. In
the tub itself, we first put a shower stool, and then a shower
bench. A walk-in shower would have been easier to deal with,
but you deal with what you have.

So, she had clearly made an irreversible step down. My
mistake then was to imagine that she would remain on that
level, that the accommodation would work. Of course, it
did, but only for a while. The cane would be discarded in
favor of a walker. Since Carol was still ambulatory and even
thought of taking walks outside along the road, we opted
for a four-wheel model, which included a seat, the idea being
that during those planned outdoor walks, she could sit down
for a rest. In the house, I could sometimes save her the difficulty of walking from point A to B by having her sit on
the walker's seat while I pushed her as though she were in a
wheelchair. At this stage, when we went grocery shopping, I
would leave the walker in the car, get the shopping cart, and
she would use that as a kind of walker.

That notion of outdoor walks turned out to be unrealistic.
I'm not sure, at this point, if we ever succeeded in getting
up to the road. My memory tells me that on one or two occasions, we made it up the driveway and onto the grass, which

the four wheels of the walker were supposed to handle. But that did not last long. She took a more sudden drop onto the next step, and the wheeled walker had to be abandoned in favor of a four-legged pick up and put down variety such as the one her mother used. I added two wheels to the front legs and cut off tennis balls for the rear so it would slide. It didn't take long for her to get the hang of that setup. She stayed on that step of the down staircase for a while, but it was significantly farther down from the starting point, which I would mark as pre-dementia.

I can't be precise in drawing my imagined graph. It seems to me that for some time, she managed with that walker. But then the stairs started to cause anxiety, and I installed two grab bars on the second floor where she would step onto the stairs. In a similar way, our old farmhouse offered steps going out of the house into an entrance room and then again into the garage, and so I attached grab bars at those doorways.

With these accommodations, while she was doing decently well in the house, on the occasions we went somewhere—to a doctor's appointment, or to the restaurant where we usually ate once a week—the walker was proving to be a bit troublesome getting from the car to the building, through the door, and to somewhere inside.

We had already obtained a handicap placard for the car and now bought a transport chair. I would load it into the trunk of the car and then use it to access whatever building we were entering. In the restaurant, she would remain seated in the transport chair at the table. At home, we would, for a while, perform the same strategy of her going to the dinner table in the transport chair.

The transport chair now sits idly at the foot of the stairs because Carol began to have serious problems ascending those steps. I would get behind her and encourage her to go up. For a while that approach was working, but not for very long. After a time, she would panic at some point going up, leading to increasingly untenable situations where she would insist on sitting down where there was nothing good to land on. Standing behind her, I could ease her down into a sitting position and then help her back to her feet. She could then be encouraged to resume the upward direction.

Until she wasn't so to be encouraged, and we abandoned the idea of her going upstairs, the state we are now in and have been for some time as I write this.

And then some weeks ago, another big downward step as her panicked fear of falling deepened to the point where she no longer can stand up, never mind walk. This inability is not due to muscular weakness. Her legs remain quite strong. But her head convinces her that she is falling.

That level has steadied for the while.

Throughout this period, I harbored the fond hope that the downward motion could be changed, that she would again climb the steps, or failing that, that she would again stand and use the walker, or failing that, that she would stand long enough to pivot onto the chair.

Of course, that did not happen.

The movement charting her condition is a one-way highway.

One with no place for U-turns, or off-ramps.

I look back over my imagined graph, an object associated with each dip, each object intended to counteract the effects of the inevitable decline. The odd thing is that at each point, these objects were like stations on a railroad track, but not any station, more like a depot or destination. In my mind, I now realize I concentrated on the temporary pause in the movement, thinking of it as a place where this hideous journey would stop.

Foolish, of course. In hindsight, blindingly so. But at each station, I imagined we were detraining, picking up our luggage, and moving into our new quarters. You see, I can hear myself saying to myself, those new grab bars I so cunningly installed have now enabled her to deal with the stairs, or navigate her way through those pesky doorways.

And each time when this false comfort was dashed, and

we were back on that cursed train, we would approach a new station, and I would provide the necessary item to get us there, a new walker, or a shower bench, or a transport chair, and repeat the fantasy, and we would detrain and stay there for at least a while.

And each time that hope was dashed much sooner than I expected, and we were back on the track heading to some final destination, where at long last we would be at trip's end.

Where our journey will end.

Fix-it

Just back from town for weekly grocery shopping. At the butcher shop one of the clerks asked after Carol. We always used to food shop together, and this person hadn't realized that I had been coming by myself for some time. When I explained why Carol was not, and would not be, accompanying me, this clerk did what it seems everybody does in that situation: she referenced her grandmother whom she said, she had seen, but had not been seen by, for fifteen years. Such a response, I suppose, is a way of sharing. The first few times somebody so shared, it was mildly comforting, saying together we belong to this group of suffering human beings.

I confess, now, it has become a touch annoying. It is sad to see the cognitive deterioration of a grandparent. But it is not unusual. To see the same but much earlier deterioration in your spouse is just of a different order.

I've heard that men often try to fix problems. In relationship advice expositions of this tendency, men are encouraged to just listen to the woman's account of what is troubling her. I saw an amusing video to this effect posted online in which the woman is describing a discomfort she feels in her head. When the camera shifts to the man's perspective, we see that the woman has a nail in her forehead. The man tries to point out that fact. She continues talking about the discomfort. He listens, perplexed. The title of the video is "It's Not About the Nail."

I am not interested in the relationship implications of this gender analysis. And I have no idea whether it is, in fact, true that males feel compelled to fix things while females desire an empathetic listener. Dealing with such hypotheses is well beyond my pay grade. But what I can say without hesitation is that whatever the case might be for my male compatriots, I have that trait.

I want things to work as they are supposed to. If they don't, I become irritated. I try to make them behave. These attempts at fixing mechanical problems can be problematic but usually not fatally so. I am persistent enough, intelligent enough, and wary of not doing anything stupid enough, to generally manage to fix things rather than do further damage. That combination of limited natural talent and decent intelligence indicates why, had I continued with my original college plan to become an engineer, I would have been a mediocre one, forever swimming upstream.

Did not get much writing on this on my last session. Life intervened, most significantly by introducing Carol's stomach to something upsetting, resulting in vomiting and diarrhea for the better part of an afternoon.

She's better now, and I have just made my way, with some difficulty, back from our mailbox. On this rural stretch of road, all the mailboxes are on one side to accommodate the carrier's route. Our mailbox happens to be across the road. That can be a bit of an issue in the winter, but there is no snow yet. On the other hand, the leaf peepers are out in full force, driving up and down the Peninsula as the leaves, particularly on the maples, begin to turn. We are nowhere near full color, and yet I had to wait several minutes each way of my crossing, and even with the wait, I was obliged to hustle. I can see what's coming from the south for a decent distance. From the north, however, traffic comes roaring up and over the crest of a hill. This road is a state highway with a 55 mile per hour speed limit that is often exceeded. A little inattention, as for example if I were to be looking at the envelopes in my hand as I head back to our house, and I would be roadkill.

I will try to pick up the thread where I last left it before Carol's illness.

My most recent fix-it project involved our fairly new dishwasher. As with so many contemporary products, this otherwise sturdy appliance relies on little pieces of plastic in what can be important places. In this instance, it has decorative plastic clip-on pieces at the end of the track through which the rollers of the top rack slide. The job of these pieces is to stop the rack from riding off the track. After a wash cycle one day I found a plastic piece from the left side track on the floor of the tub.

As many times as I popped that piece back on, it would not hold. I observed how the one on the right was positioned, duplicated it for the one on the left, and maybe it would remain where it belongs for a couple of washes. Then, thinking I had finally fixed the problem, I would slide the top rack out to put something at the back of it, only to have the rack continue past its end and dangle without support.

At first, I simply resolved that this matter, particularly in light of the other more pressing complexities of my life, was simply not worth my attention. And yet, I could not tolerate the fact that this part of the machine was not operating as it should. I recalled how a repair technician solved a similar problem on a previous machine, and I came up with an answer.

I fashioned a new stop for the track, using a four-inch plastic cable tie threaded through openings on the end of the track so that it would block the wheel where the plastic used to perform that function.

The repair has worked, and I feel a little surge of satisfaction every time I roll that top rack out. The thing is again working as it should.

I find it difficult to leave problems alone. I will persist and apply my limited mechanical aptitude until I find a solution, or failing that, eventually cry uncle and call in a professional.

I am facing such an annoyance now with my watch, which

has a little window through which a number corresponding to the day of the month appears. The mechanism that causes whatever this number is inscribed on to turn to the next date has somehow gotten out of whack. I'm guessing that the mechanism has to be lined up in such a way as to ignore the sweep of the minute hand past noon, and then turn some kind of wheel to expose the next number when the minute hand goes by twelve midnight.

However, it does not quite do that. Rather, it either turns too early, so that the new number shows up after noon, or too late, so that the old number remains after midnight until noon the next day. I have tried to fix this malfunction by using the adjusting stem that manually changes the number when it is pulled halfway out so as to be able to work around all those months that do not have thirty-one days. But no matter when I make the adjustment, such as turning to the new number right after midnight, the problem returns, unchastened and bold.

Clearly, I can't fix it. Perhaps a watch expert can, but in spite of my irritation, this is just not worth the effort now. So, I will live with the fact that as I look at my watch at this moment, it insists that it is the 22nd when I know full well it is the 21st.

Whether or not I am exhibiting a typical, or perhaps an exaggerated, version of the male fix-it mentality, I respond to most problems with an urge to set things right. In my professional life as a college administrator, this trait was probably useful. As a writer, and teacher of writing, it underscores my purposeful emphasis on rewriting. And, as I have indicated, in my personal life, matters large and small induce the same response.

How then do I fix Carol? How to restore the wheels in her head so that they line up properly again and mesh as they are supposed to?

There is no place to fasten a tie to stop her thoughts from sliding off the track.

I cannot make that repair any more than I can get my watch to function properly again.

To fix my watch I have the option to take it into town to a jeweler.

But there is no expert repair shop that will restore Carol to her wonderfully working self.

That failure produces in me an emotion laced with anger, frustration, and above all, a constant and deepening sadness.

Two Worlds

Another rainy fall day. Turning colors on trees becoming more vibrant and worth a drive up the Peninsula to witness, but rain has dampened the leaf peepers' enthusiasm today, so I made an uneventful crossing to our mailbox, only to retrieve one thin piece of bulk mail, which I tossed into our waste bin on my way back into the house. Carol was fidgeting and thinking she was falling because her legs were dangling off the sofa. I repositioned her, and she is now lapsing into her afternoon drowse. I'll take the opportunity to see what thoughts are looking for a way out of my mind.

Here is our morning routine.

I rouse from sleep on my half of our sectional sofa and see to Carol's hygienic needs, then I empty the dishwasher, feed and let out the dog, and then prepare Carol's breakfast, usually melon chunks or a banana, toast, a breakfast sausage, and juice. When she is settled down from all of that, including encouraging her to swallow her morning meds, I go upstairs to shower and dress for the day.

That trip upstairs always brings a wave of sadness, nothing intense because it is replicated daily, but strong enough to remind me of how different my life, or should I say, our lives, have become. Entering our upstairs, I cross the border into another country. Even the dog, who nearly always positions herself in my vicinity, seems to recognize that I am leaving our common living space and contents herself with settling on the first landing if she ventures up the steps at all. Only when I spend a decent interval in my office does the dog decide to figure out what has happened to me.

Granted all of that, our upstairs still forcibly reminds me of the then of our lives rather than the now. In our bedroom are our two dressers and our two clothing closets. Because of the configuration of this room in our old farmhouse, there is not space for two night tables. The one we have, an antique little cabinet we purchased from the antique shop halfway to town, sits between the bed and the doorway. Before I installed our set of cordless instruments, we only had one wired phone upstairs, located in my office in the adjacent room. Since I was the usual phone answerer—probably because of my many years of having a phone on my work office desk—even before Carol's deterioration, I positioned myself on the side of the bed nearest the doorway so when the phone rang, I would roll out of bed and stumble into my office to answer it. When we got the cordless phone, I put it on the nightstand next to my side of the bed.

For years it was thus, with Carol on the other side of the bed. We both liked to read at night, so I used the nightstand to hold whatever book I was working through. Because there was no corresponding nightstand on the other side of the bed, I put a short shelf over the headboard to hold Carol's books. However, at the beginning of her difficulties, she began to experience trouble navigating from that side of the bed, around it, and then out the doorway, across the hall, to the bathroom.

As a result, we switched sides. I still answered the phone when necessary by reaching across her. She piled her reading material on the nightstand next to the phone. Still sitting there is an issue of Scientific American. Every day as I sit on the bed putting on my socks reminds me again of the scope and variety of her interests, frankly a good deal wider than mine, although mine perhaps run a little deeper.

When I exit the shower, I take my towel from the rack. Her towel, now long unused, remains hanging on the rack. When I reach into the storage space a previous owner fashioned into a closet by installing shelves and folding doors in front of them, I see that my items are housed only on the top shelf while hers occupy the others. In the shower itself is the corner caddy on which standing upside down still is the bottle of her hair conditioner.

Its companion bottle containing the shampoo is now on a shelf in the downstairs bathroom near the couch in the living room. She had always taken very good care of her luxuriously thick hair. The combination shampoo/conditioner set was of especially good quality, which I would order online as necessary.

That the two bottles are now divided upstairs and down, the latter being administered occasionally by one aide, the former not at all, underscores the then and now that we are living through.

Two bottles, one in each of the worlds, past and present.

The constant tug back and forth, the past muscling itself into our present.

Hope

It's either cool or cold today according to your frame of mind. I won't choose. It is somewhere in between. No sun and a steady drizzling rain that might develop into something more significant. Reports of street flooding in town, but no danger of that here, sitting as we do atop a hill.

A new physical therapist will be here soon to do an evaluation to determine if she will undertake another round. The goal will be more modest than in past therapeutic efforts. This time we are looking to get Carol back on her feet, literally. Resuming walking may be beyond the range of possible outcomes.

I am also aware that part of the need for an evaluation at this juncture is to project the benefits of the therapy so as to convince insurance to pay for it.

In any event, I am snatching a little writing time now, sitting across from Carol in our living room. After being quite talkative—although I cannot say about what—she is about to start her afternoon drowse.

A realization has occurred to me. As I write, I find myself expressing myself, on occasion, in a light-hearted manner that is most definitely at odds with our situation. This should not surprise me. I have always during life's dark moments sought a little humor to lift the gloom. Doing so is not a conscious decision. It is how I am wired.

If I try to analyze myself to explain myself to myself, I recall hearing somewhere a handwriting expert suggest that an individual's basic personality can be revealed in the strokes of pen or pencil. Even as I write that I wonder if this kind of expertise is becoming a quaint relic as more and more people only tap out their thoughts on a keyboard rather than inscribe them on paper.

Be that as it may, we still sign things like credit card receipts, and perhaps that will continue to provide a sufficient basis for what that long-ago expert had to say. What has remained in my memory was the assertion that if the handwriting literally had an upward tilt to it, it reflects a core optimism. My handwriting, as miserable as it is, has such a tilt, most noticeable in how I cross the *t* in my name. I do so with a longer line than is necessary and with a strong upward tilt from left to right. I even feel a bit of a rush of energy when I make that line, which I do after I have scrawled the other letters of my name.

So it would appear, if that expert's ideas have any validity, that I have a solid core of optimism in my emotional makeup.

I feel that is correct.

I also know that optimism seems totally out of place in our current situation. On the one hand, it is. On the other, an irrational optimism stiffens my resistance to yielding to this awful disease.

It will defeat us. I know that. But not without one hell of a fight.

And on some level, I believe Carol shares that determination. She was never deterred from going after anything she wanted or to lose what she had.

I do think that even now, on some level, that strength of purpose remains.

She does not want to give in.

Settled into my writing chair in the living room across from Carol sleeping on the sofa. Usually, she does not fall asleep as early or soundly as she has done tonight. I think she was knocked out by the session with the physical and occupational therapists this morning.

I did my grocery shopping this afternoon and needed a rest before making supper for us. On shopping days it's always frozen dinners. Carol's is lasagna and she eats it with a good appetite. For me, a Hungry-Man dinner.

Dog is knocked out also, but that is normal.

Today Carol worked with her third physical therapist as well as her third occupational therapist.

I thought we had moved beyond the reach of both kinds of therapy. We had started with occupational therapy a couple of years ago shortly after Carol's treatment for breast cancer was completed. At that time, we were working on her restoring her handwriting, which had been a thing of pride and beauty. But after chemo, she could not manage to write on a straight line or start at the left margin.

In my ignorance then, I thought this problem could be, and would be, fixed.

Of course, the problem only got worse. We moved on to the first physical therapist, who concentrated on exercises to strengthen her trunk. When that therapist thought she had done what she could, she left us with a sheet showing how to do each of the exercises, along with a pedal device with which Carol was to continue strengthening her legs.

More or less at the same time, we worked with the second occupational therapist with the goal of restoring Carol's skill on the keyboard. She had been an excellent typist.

I thought, naively, that muscle memory would kick in and fingers would again find the keys as they used to.

Of course, that didn't happen, any more than the piano lessons we signed up for restored her ability on that kind of keyboard.

When her mobility difficulties worsened, we worked with the second physical therapist, with the goal of getting her able to go up the stairs.

I've written about that failed effort.

I did not see much point in continuing to work with either variety of therapy.

But our nurse practitioner, observing Carol's inability to get off the couch and recognizing that she was more than strong enough so to do, suggested we try yet again. I agreed, so the third physical therapist came last week and asked if she could return with an occupational therapist to see if the two could combine their efforts.

That is what happened today.

With a degree of success.

They managed to get Carol on her feet, and then also into her travel chair for a little movement around the house. These feats were accomplished in spite of Carol's spirited, and occasionally profane, resistance.

As I witness their working with Carol, I felt a little stirring of hope.

Maybe, just maybe, in spite of the heavy weight of the downward movement of the disease, that movement could be stayed, and even to a small, but not insignificant degree, reversed.

A great success would be to get Carol back on her feet. Perhaps even to walk a little.

Is that too much to hope for?

My core optimism answers, in spite of all evidence to the contrary, in the affirmative.

A Train to Somewhere/Early Signs of Trouble Ahead

Just back from walking through a steady, light drizzle across the road to the mailbox where I found nothing much of interest besides the latest Smithsonian, one of the magazines we both enjoyed, I for the history, Carol for the science.

It seems as though the sun has only made token appearances for the past couple of weeks, just enough to remind us of its existence. Otherwise, we are enduring gloomy, rainy weather, only brightened by the fall colors of the leaves that will before long be brown and on the ground.

It is hard to be cheery on days such as these.

I feel like I am on a train heading toward an unknown destination and looking back to the station where I can see a figure, a woman, standing on the platform. It is not clear whether her eyes are directed at the train and, if so, whether she will wave or just turn away.

She stands, motionless. Her arm does not come up.

That is Carol.

Until now, for the most part, I have strained to hold on to her as though her disease was taking her away from me. And, in truth, it is doing just that by loosening her grip on the now while moving more and more into the then of that part of her life still stored in her long-term memory.

But I am just now recognizing my own movement away. It is not something I willed myself to do. Quite the contrary. Yet, just a little while ago, I saw an old film camera on the bookcase in our bedroom. For some reason, as I picked it up sadness descended on me with an almost physical intensity. My eyes moistened in response.

The person who used that camera to indulge her love of

photography, a manifestation of her highly visual relation-ship to the world, that person rarely focuses her eyes on any-thing, and instead responds to the visions her brain manu-factures for her from who knows what source, be it memory, or imagination, or some combination of both.

I imagine her disease has put her on that railroad station platform.

It is I who, inevitably, will have to move forward.

Somewhere.

Somehow.

I recognize that this down mood will not last. I will not let it. I never permit myself to wallow in self-pity for very long. Writing is something of an antidote. And then I recall that slight basis for hope prompted by what is probably the overly optimistic assessment of the therapists that they feel some progress has been made, and more is possible.

I permit myself to buy into that proposition.

If the train won't reverse itself, perhaps I can get off.

Late Thursday evening after a hectic, social day, my weekly lunch, then dinner with brother and sister-in-law while nephew stayed with Carol, between these events the arrival of a new caregiver relief person, who turned out fine. The lunch crew now includes two retired sociology professors, a retired social worker, and an engineer. Con-versation includes some politics—we all lean left—along with local news and personal items. Supper talk more family centric as it should be.

Had the occasion to go through Carol's wallet looking for her insurance card. Some sad reminders in the scraps of paper therein. On those, various notes and reminders writ-ten in her beautiful hand, of which she was so rightly proud, and which I wondered at, given my nearly unreadable scrawl.

Too tired last night to continue, so picking it up here.

I am finding as I work on this journal, and in so doing, look

more closely at ordinary things that there were clues point-
ing toward where we are now, but they were seemingly not
significant and easily explained away.

Among those papers in her wallet was one that listed the
three steps necessary to unlock her mother's front door. It
has a keyless lock. To open it, you turn a pointer to three
numbers in a certain order, and it opens. The sequence is not
that hard to remember, but Carol had written it down.

Innocent enough, perhaps, but it was only one such paper
reminder in her wallet. Another was a list of the telephone
numbers of her family. These are the kinds of numbers it
would not be uncommon to have memorized.

Still, nothing that dramatic in these pieces of paper, just
a bit of an indicator that she did not rely on her memory
in these cases. But then I found another piece of paper on
which was written her own cell phone number. That's a little
more unusual.

It also reminds me that she never really mastered her
phone.

Or the microwave.

Or the computer beyond word processing and emailing.
Never did much on the Internet.

It is hard to explain these difficulties occurring in a
woman who was quite at home with machines, tractors and
other farm equipment, cars, and such like. And a woman
who had the manual dexterity to play the piano and type at
an impressive rate.

Perhaps her brain is just wired in a certain way, as all
brains are. I'm sure that is part of the answer. But perhaps
these difficulties can also be traced to the very incipient
stages of what became her disease.

I see some memory issues in the notes to herself in her
wallet. Those same issues might also explain her replicating
filing systems by setting up the same files in several different places. Material relevant to our daughter is located in
three or four different filing drawers.

Is that a memory issue?

I don't know.

If it is, it did not prevent her from being a steady A student through her education culminating in her law degree.

What I can say is that for the first sixty some odd years of her life whatever these issues were did not prevent her from functioning on a very high level.

Then she got breast cancer.

And chemotherapy.

Thereafter, her early onset dementia, which might have been barely discernible, made its presence known with force and effect. In my mind, I have clear before chemo and after chemo pictures, and they are dramatically different.

I can only conclude, and various medical professionals have agreed, that the chemo accelerated the progress of the disease so that she might not have reached where she is now for another ten or more years.

Whenever I think about this, I have difficulty containing my anger. The tumor was tiny. It had not spread. Only because advances in biochemistry made it possible for an analysis of the tumor to indicate that it was of an aggressive type pointed toward similarly aggressive treatment. Had we known that the effect of the chemo might accelerate her dementia, we no doubt would have opted for its removal, no chemo, and a wait-and-see approach.

Her medical records must have indicated that she had already been sent for neuropsychological testing, which showed minor impairment. We knew this and thought it was something to be dealt with down the road.

We did not know, nor were we warned, that chemo might accelerate her speed down that road.

The oncologist just followed her usual protocol for such cases.

And there it was, and here we are.

Betwixt Then and Now / Within Sight of Land

Spent the morning dealing with issues related to the historical society website for which I used to be the webmaster. The last part of that term is not to be taken literally: I was hugely assisted in that capacity by our daughter Danielle. The society, as an act of mercy, has taken that responsibility away from me, and in so doing contracted with a new web hosting service. That, in turn, involves removing me from the domain name, and doing that runs into password issues, all of which we managed to straighten out.

It always feels good to problem solve, especially now when the problem has nothing to do with Carol. However, soon after that issue was taken care of, I confronted another insurance issue, this one involving payment for physical and occupational therapy. An hour's work with the physical therapist who used to be a case manager in insurance and can talk insurancese seems to have solved that problem.

The physical therapist is the only one of the professionals I have been dealing with who seems wholeheartedly to agree with my decision, thus far, to keep Carol at home with me. Other views from family, friends, and professionals range from the I should think of myself school to those who don't take a position but respect what I am doing to others whose focus is only on Carol and what can be done within the parameters of my decision.

In truth, there is no good answer. That seems to be the rule in all matters related to the course of this disease.

My present situation offers substantial pluses and minuses. On the plus side, and in keeping with the thread I have been developing, having Carol here with me offers a stasis between the then and now. Except for largely now discarded items such as the walkers and travel chair scattered about the house, our living environment hasn't changed much. And, of course, her continued presence, especially when we sleep near each other, reinforces the continuity of the then into the now.

But I am sort of living alone since we do not really interact in meaningful ways as once we did. I have lived alone at various times in my life, most particularly as a point of comparison, after my separation from my first wife. But in that situation, I was free to live as I pleased, go where I please, while maintaining my professional obligations, going to work and socializing when and with whom I chose.

Now, though, my activities are circumscribed, conducted only at times when I have arranged for caregiver relief. So, in a sense I am living alone while not living, strictly speaking, alone. I serve Carol food but eat by myself. For the evening meal, I make two place settings at the dining room table as if for both of us but take Carol's plate and silverware over to the couch where I help her eat her dinner. Then I sit by myself at the dining room table with no one to talk to, my companion the dog at my feet ever hopeful for a piece of food to drop off the table to her.

Breakfast runs the same way although for some reason I have mine in the kitchen. Maybe I do so to be near the Keurig and/or the dog's dish waiting to be filled. And, of course, I must retrieve the local paper without which it would be impossible for me to eat my breakfast.

Lunch is a hit and miss affair for both of us, but in practice comes closest to accurately illustrating my immersion into the now. Carol often is not hungry for lunch. I sometimes skip it as well or grab something quick like a cup of yogurt. When Carol does express an interest, I bring her a protein bar or a sandwich. Only very rarely do I eat lunch more or less at the same time.

These mealtime scenarios exemplify what I am talking about. Lunch is the most accurate representation of our now reality. Breakfast and supper, on the other hand, hover betwixt and between then and now, beginning with the pretense of a shared meal, quickly dropped, and followed by the cold reality of now, as we take our sustenance separately.

Traverse City, and the peninsula north of it where we live, have a large, perhaps disproportionate, number of permanent older residents. Some are retirees who have come to enjoy the arts and culture the small city has to offer along with the beautiful landscape of water and hills. Others are retirees of a different sort, the older generation of the farming community, who see no reason, as many of their peers in other places do, to move to Florida or Arizona or other warm weather havens. Some of these do winter in those places while the hardier ones stay home and deal with the cold and the snow.

The point is that whenever I go out after the tourists have left, the odds of seeing folks sixty years old and above are strikingly high. In the grocery store today, I was walking behind a white-haired woman pushing her cart, accompanied by a middle-aged woman, who appeared to be her daughter, or at least a close relative. Together, they were filling their cart while discussing the choices available on the shelves. The older one could easily have been in her eighties. She walked with care, but she walked. And she was fully engaged in the shopping.

In the same store, I bumped into an old friend of Carol's, a woman with whom she had worked on various local history projects. That woman was a descendant of one of the original farming families. Her intense interest in her own family, and by extension, local history, led her to me when I was working on my historical novel set here and based on a sensational 1895 murder case. She and Carol became fast friends.

She was there shopping with her husband. We chatted a bit, and I filled them in on Carol's condition. We discovered we were all in our middle seventies.

The first woman was in her eighties.

All of us doing our weekly grocery shopping.

What's wrong with this picture?

Carol is not yet sixty-five and will never again join with me in this mundane chore.

And I feel profoundly cheated.

Cheated in a particular way that Stephen Crane wonderfully presented in his short story "The Open Boat," in which he writes, "When it occurs to a man that nature does not regard him as important . . . he at first wishes to throw bricks at the temple, and he hates deeply the fact that there are no bricks and no temples. . . . Thereafter he knows the pathos of his situation."

Thus, Crane describes the thoughts of a man in a lifeboat, who contemplates the real possibility that he and the others with him in the boat could well die, killed by the indifferent force of nature, the ocean on which like a tiny cork they bob within sight of land they cannot reach.

That is how I feel. I want to strike out at something but can find no target except the indifferent force of dementia.

Carol's disease substitutes for Crane's nature, both violently hostile, and yet indifferent, seemingly unaware, of the damage they inflict.

This train of thought brings me to another piece of Crane's writing, one of his bitingly acerbic short poems:

A man said to the universe:

"Sir, I exist!"

"However," replied the universe,

"The fact has not created in me

A sense of obligation."

Yes, Carol and I exist.

Bobbing on the indifferent waves in our own little boat within sight of the unreachable and slowly receding land.

Changing

Just back from a trip to my desktop in my office upstairs to work on Quicken, which is not on my laptop. Coming back down to my usual nighttime chair across from Carol on the couch, I notice that the dog stayed in her bed instead of following me wherever I go as she usually does. She seems to have decided it's not worth the energy to go upstairs with me.

A difficult day with Carol because she was not in the here and now for much of the time. Instead, she appeared to be fixed on whatever auditory hallucinations were occupying her brain. There are two results from times such as these. The first is they are distracting; the second is they augur a substantive change.

As for the first result, it is in a minor way irritating. It's as though there's an animated conversation occurring that on the level of noise is distracting when I am trying to read, do my puzzles, or work on the laptop. I grew up in an environment that conditioned me to ignore distracting noise. I rode the New York subways doing my assigned reading oblivious to the crowds shuffling on and off through opening and closing doors, or the screech of steel wheels on steel tracks, or the garbled voice coming through the speaker announcing the upcoming stations.

I think I have lost some of that hard shell.

Sometimes in her internal conversations, Carol actually screams. At other times, she yells out "OW!" as if suddenly in pain. If I ask what is hurting her, the best I get is some vague gesture.

In any case, her expressions of pain, or need, or anger demand my attention and take me away from whatever else I am doing. For the most part, that is of no consequence, but occasionally I might be on the phone dealing with some issue, such as possible credit card fraud, or quite often an insurance billing problem, that I must attend to.

The second result of this kind of behavior disconnected from the present moment is more troubling because it leads to a more important shift. On the immediate level, as much as I know in a rational way that she is arguing with, sometimes cursing out, an unknown person in her head, I respond as though the words were directed at me. That is a perfectly plausible consequence. We have been living together for thirty-five years. I naturally respond to her voice as though she is saying something to me. Worse, sometimes, in a sense, she is talking to me because she is addressing the Steve in her head, and uses his name, so reasonably I hear that and accept, for the moment, that she is actually conversing with, or as the case might be, yelling at me.

Today, there was a great deal of that kind of activity.

And it led me to a sudden unexpected, and unwanted, revelation.

I am changing.

I have been tracking the changes in Carol, as though I have remained as I had been.

But it occurred to me today with considerable force that my attitude toward our situation also moves along its own track. And that track will take me away from my attachment to the then and move me toward the now and past that to some sort of future.

This hit home this afternoon when I was down in the basement to bring up the storm doors to insert them in place of the screen doors. While in the furnace room, where these doors are stored, my eyes caught a faux leather, open box that contained a few CDs and framed pictures. I'm always looking for music, so I first paid attention to the CDs. They didn't interest me much. I didn't recognize the artists or the music. But then I examined the photos. They were from our daughter's early years. There standing at water's edge of some beach was my beautiful, and most important, glowingly happy Carol.

That image pierced my let's get this job done mood. That Carol is so not here, not even remotely. Physically she has not changed that much. In fact, her age has treated her gently.

But the woman whose smile glowed on that beach with our young daughter is no more.

And that intense feeling of loss, I realized, is moving me, however reluctantly, away from my grip on the used to be.

I am not happy about it.

But it is probably a necessary separation.

Back from an appointment in town, I am sitting on a not terribly comfortable chair in front of a window in the Peninsula Community Library through which in the background, past a path flanked by weeds and the tops of trees rising from a deep dip in the land, I can catch a glimpse of the blue waters of the western arm of Grand Traverse Bay. The library is housed in the same building as the local elementary school, the same school Carol attended so many years ago. I have come here today because my caregiver relief person has arrived, and this is my opportunity to get out for a while and forget my here and now responsibilities.

I am reminded that Carol enjoyed coming to this library to do her writing although we had set up several writing stations for her at home. But still she often chose to pack her laptop into her attaché case and drive the six or seven miles to the library. I believe she was seeking company. That is a bit of a contradiction, but one that makes sense. She was easily distracted, thus the appeal of her barn studio office in our outer building where there would only be a little occasional noise from the road or tractors across the way in the orchards. On the other hand, however, she loved being among people. In some ways, the library offered, I suppose, a workable compromise: mostly quiet but people there for as much interaction as she wanted.

I now have a fuller understanding of that compromise. I

am not nearly as distractible as she, nor do I crave company as she did. For most of my life, where I worked made little difference. When able, such as in my own house, I generally would have music playing although after a while when deep into my writing I would no longer hear it. Even now as I get into this piece the background noise from the kids in the library doesn't really intrude into my consciousness.

But there is a huge difference in how I think about my workstation now. I live so much alone, even when Carol is fifteen feet away from me. I thought about that fact as I drove into town. I always, now, drive alone. Maybe I should start taking the dog for company, as I see many single drivers do. In anticipating a long road trip to New York in March, I realize I have not done one of those by myself in many years. I love to drive, and I will have my music, but nobody to talk to.

Before I left for town today, I found myself talking to the caregiver relief person about personal matters having little direct connection to her responsibilities with Carol. I mentioned that I would stop at the library on the way back, this to inform her that I would not be home much before my time was up. But then I explained that while at the library, besides doing some writing, I was going to start researching possible choices for my next lease car, which I will have to choose in a couple of months.

I was happy to have a little conversation even with a woman who is little more than a stranger, the kind of conversation I would routinely have had with Carol. In fact, she was the reason I began leasing cars when she was unhappy with the '95 Bonneville I was driving, then about twelve years old and beginning to show some signs of age-related problems.

At that time, each of us had our own car. That had been true in New York. We bought an all-wheel drive Subaru Forrester to be Carol's car when we moved to the snows of northern Michigan, and after a while here we replaced the Bonneville with a leased Nissan Altima.

I know the registrations for each car were in the name of

the primary driver. Registrations renew according to the birthday of the registrant, and so the Subaru came up for renewal on Carol's birthday, the Nissan on mine.

The titles were in both our names. When we sold Carol's Subaru to our niece because it had become clear that Carol would not be driving any more, I signed over the title paper for her. Carol's name is still on the Nissan title.

If Carol were now aware of these kinds of matters, she no doubt would want her name on the new lease car or added to the title should I decide to buy the present one. She did not give up driving easily. She would surrender her ownership in some form of a vehicle even more reluctantly.

I have to do that for her.

And I record these thoughts in the same library where a time ago she chose to come to work, and where I now appreciate the incidental social interaction offered to me here. I could write at home in my office, but I feel that would be a waste of my respite time, on the one hand, and I have a felt need to be out and among people on the other.

Like Carol did.

In a perverse and ironic sense, in some ways such as this, I now understand Carol better than before.

I could thank her disease for that gift.

But I think I will pass.

Long View

Carol sleeping noisily on the sofa, this Thanksgiving night. The day, predictably, was quiet, folks everywhere celebrating the holiday in their own way. In the early afternoon, the pastor of the Methodist church Carol sometimes attended, called up to say someone would be by to drop off two dinners for us. This kind gesture was not at all unexpected. There was more food than we could handle, given Carol's diminished appetite, so later in the afternoon, I heated up one of the two dinners and will save the second for another time.

Otherwise, Carol, whose stomach has been acting up, drowsed on and off, and I watched a lot of football.

Our daughter Danielle is planning a visit next month around the holidays. I have encouraged her to read this journal in preparation as she has not seen her mother in almost a year. She said that she has read parts of it.

But that is not enough.

Nothing, really, is enough.

I am concerned as to how she will handle the shock that awaits her. It is possible that Carol will not recognize her, as extraordinary a statement as that is. I have concluded that Carol's siblings have stayed away because they find it difficult to see her like this. That is, perhaps, a kinder way of looking at their seeming indifference, but maybe a more accurate one. They, of course, grew up with her, knew her for the bright vital person she was, and saw her that way during the years since we moved here.

For Danielle, as her daughter, I can only imagine the emotions will run much deeper and stronger. Mother and daughter were very close through all the growing-up years. Danielle has Asperger's and Carol, long before the diagnosis, sensed that there was a problem and was protective. In spite of the autism, Danielle has managed quite well, got her bachelor's degree, found employment, lived in Cleveland for her first job, and is now working in Minnesota and completing an associate degree in programming.

As she reached college age and now through her years of employment, she and I have grown closer, and her relationship with Carol is not as tight as it had been. But still, there is a lot of history between them. I think of their shared love of cats. Danielle has always had one or more cats in her apartments. They both enjoyed the Cat Who books.

Carol brought her up to be a strong woman, and that, I am sure, has enabled Danielle to overcome the obstacles posed by her autism.

She will need that strength as she confronts her mother's diminished capacity.

She and I were texting this evening while she was still at work, talking about driving versus flying to get here, and that led to conversation about cars, and what I was thinking of doing when my current lease expires in a couple of months.

After we were through exchanging messages, I was looking at the app on my phone. I saw that it offered a link to pictures, those I had sent her, and those she had sent me. I looked through these images. Among them were a couple of pictures of our rescue Golden Retriever, and from Danielle's end some scenes of cloud formations that intrigued her. She shares her mother's keen visual sense and love of photography. Other images sometimes served a practical purpose, such as one I sent showing her what baseboard heating looks like so she could tell me if that is what was in her apartment, so I could guess at the source of her heating problem.

But most striking and heart wrenching for me was a pair of images from August of 2016. One of them is of Carol sitting at our kitchen table, with a little smile on her face, and waving. I couldn't remember the context for this one until I saw its companion sent from Danielle, showing her sitting at her workstation and also waving. I remember now that these photos arose out of a phone call as a kind of still picture version of Skype.

What struck me is that Carol is sitting up at the table, something she no longer can do. I believe, if I look closely at the picture, she is sitting in the transport chair. I must have wheeled her in that to the table.

Now, I cannot without great difficulty get her into that chair.

The picture was shot sixteen months ago.

Checking my calendar, I see that those pictures were taken just a few days after we returned from our visit to see Danielle in Minnesota, a trip of about six hundred miles each way, involving stops in motels.

I cannot get Carol out of the living room, much less into the car.

Danielle saw her mother here last January, when we were still able to go out to eat.

We will not be able to do that this time.

Thinking about all this is so painful. Living with Carol from day to day, I don't often take the longer view that I just did.

It's like picking off a scab to see that the skin below is still raw.

Another almost winter day, no sun, a little snow, altogether depressing weather compounded by it being Saturday when it seems I am on my own little island while the rest of the world goes about its business. Tried to get worked up about Michigan playing Ohio State in college football, but with limited success. I've never been that interested in college sports, coming from an area thoroughly dominated by the professional versions.

It is late afternoon. Carol is dozing, and I will start thinking about supper soon.

I have attended funerals of friends or colleagues, and a few relatives of the in-law variety, but I have never experienced, close up, the death of a loved one, with one minor exception. The exception was my maternal grandmother, who lived with us for a time before going into a nursing home where she died.

In all honesty, even though she was a close blood relative, I can't say she fits the categorization of a loved one. It's not that I was not sad when she died. I simply did not have that much of a relationship with her. From the Ukraine, she spoke little English. Or it may be she was just a quiet person. Anyway, I can only recall one thing she would say from time to time, and that is "Hay is for horses," probably prompted by hearing somebody say, "Hey..." I remember a few things about her, primarily the sour cream cookies she formed with an overturned glass and baked when she lived with us. I may be fabricating a memory when I think I recall playing Casino with her. Before she moved in with us, we would sometimes visit her in Brownsville in Brooklyn, where she lived alone in what I now understand to be straitened circumstances, but that being said, she never seemed unhappy or troubled.

Just not the sort of grandmother with whom a teenager, which is what I was when she briefly lived with us, would have formed a deep emotional bond.

My line of thought here is identifying individuals with whom I had a close, ongoing relationship when they died. I guess by close I mean both emotional depth and physical proximity. My closest adult friend, best man at my wedding to Carol, fits that category. A troubled, hugely talented individual, he lived with us for a while when his emotional life after divorce had become a train wreck. He was sleeping in his college office before we invited him to stay with us. He accepted but insisted on paying rent.

He got himself together, remarried, but then separated, and was setting up his own apartment when I got a call from his daughter asking if I knew where he was. I didn't. A little later that day another phone call told me that he had been found dead of a heart attack.

He was an Okie, and I was from Brooklyn, but we became brothers.

He died twenty or so years ago, but I can still hear the concern in his daughter's voice when she called that day.

My nuclear family members—mother, father, sister—all died in Florida while I was living in New York. I did not witness their final months, weeks, or days. In the cases of my mother and sister, their deaths were sudden. My mother had heart issues and her death, when it occurred, was not unexpected. My sister died from a freak occurrence. Not long after she died, my father was thought fit enough for coronary surgery at age eighty-six, but crushed by his daughter's death, he never really recovered from the operation. I flew down the day of the operation. Thereafter, I spoke to him on the phone but because he died before I could make another trip to Florida, I did not see him again.

All of this is the context of what I am thinking about these dark, late fall days. I am less prepared for what I am living through with Carol than otherwise I might have been. I imagine that after the death of those who were deeply involved in your life, you encounter daily reminders of who they were, most especially, as with a spouse with whom you shared living space. I recall, for example, visiting Carol's uncle in the house he lived in for so many years with his wife. Recalling those visits now, there were only a few objects that seemed to have been hers. Perhaps he had, over time, removed others, or maybe there simply were not that many clearly associated with her.

In any event, he seemed to have recovered from his grief and mourning. He could talk easily about his wife, although he did not do that very much.

I know that the sense of loss I experienced at the deaths of my parents and sister was somewhat less intense because they had not been intimately involved in my life for decades. My observation of Carol's uncle dealing with the death of the woman he had spent his whole long adult life with suggests that after a certain period of time, the sharp edge of pain fades, or transforms into something more tolerable. And one somehow turns the page.

If you're waiting for the point of all this to my situation, here it is.

Just this morning, I was doing something absolutely insignificant: putting breakfast plates into the dishwasher. As I stood there with the door of the dishwasher opened it occurred to me with disproportionate force to the trivial nature of what I was doing, that we had bought that dishwasher not that long ago, and that Carol very much wanted one with a polished steel surface.

How long, I wondered, would I be struck by these moments when I remember where or when something or other came into our lives. Not mine. But ours.

And does the fact that Carol is breathing heavily across the room from me now change those experiences for me?

She is not gone.

And yet she is going.

Here or There/Like Light
from a Distant Star

Sunday night after another long, quiet, isolated and iso-lating weekend. We are in that period between Thanksgiv-ing and Christmas when the networks, aware that people's attention is elsewhere, stop broadcasting new material. So, no Masterpiece *episodes tonight. But there was an engaging fundraiser about the Everly Brothers on PBS and a Carol Burnett retrospective on CBS. I watched the first, recorded the second, and caught the end of* Sunday Night Football.

Carol ate most of the steak dinner I prepared but is rest-less now. Some nights she slides into sleep, but tonight she seems to be fighting it. I can't imagine what is going on in her brain to cause the difference.

I find myself writing more about myself than about Carol. I believe that is because she seems to have plateaued. She is certainly no better, but neither is she worse over these last weeks. We have a kind of routine that varies only in terms of the different caregiver relief people who come. There are three now. The one who has been coming the longest is just back from her own medical leave. She gives Carol a good sponge bath and hair wash each week. One of the others came for the first time this past week while the third has been here four or five times. Each has her own personality and interacts with Carol in somewhat different ways.

I am not sure Carol is aware of these different people who come to stay with her.

Carol continues to talk to some person in her head. There seems to be a disagreement.

The physical and occupational therapists are back after

the resolution of an insurance screwup that prevented their coming. Again, as they had done before, they managed to get Carol on her feet, but only as the result of some serious effort from the two of them working together. Carol is also on an anti-vertigo medicine on the off chance that vertigo might be part of her problem. I am not optimistic but see no reason not to try that approach.

I began by saying I find myself writing about myself, and that is so because I am thinking about myself more as Carol's condition has stabilized for now. I am aware that the stability will not last, but I do not have any way of knowing its duration. What it has done, though, is given me the opportunity to kind of catch my breath and begin to think, however tentatively, about my future without her, for that is the inevitable road I am on even though I cannot know its distance.

I suppose these thoughts have been prompted in part by a newspaper clipping one of my Tuesday lunch mates gave me. It was from the Sunday *Times*, which I go through each week, but he must have dug deeper to come up with this article, which described how the north fork of Long Island is becoming the preferred destination for some city dwellers seeking a quieter lifestyle. It's an area that has some appeal for me. Although its shore front is on Long Island Sound as opposed to the ocean beaches on the south fork, it still offers miles and miles of sand and water within easy distance.

It might well be out of my price range, but perhaps not.

That is not the immediate point. We are not ready to get into those kinds of practical details.

What is the point is that I am comfortable enough where I am now. Our house is on a peninsula, so I am always near water, which seems to be a kind of constant in my life. And this primarily farming environment offers a welcome alternative to the suburban lifestyle, which I endured more than enjoyed for most of my adult life.

But I do ask myself if I want to live here without Carol. Or our daughter, who in all probability will wind up somewhere else as she thinks about a career move that will take her out of Minnesota. She never set down roots here.

Nor have I, put down roots here, that is. The physical environment is one thing. The culture is another. There is nothing wrong with Midwestern culture.

It's just not mine.

I have always said, partly in jest, and partly quite seriously, that having lived here for sixteen years, longer, in fact, in this house than others I have inhabited in my life, still, I am incompletely and imperfectly acculturated and that is as good as it is going to get.

Back east I have daughters and their families including four grandchildren and a number of very good friends and former colleagues. I do not see myself blending any more fully into Carol's family. That's not anybody's fault. We are just not that good a match. Having Carol here with me was all I needed to be comfortable. Without her, I just am not sure.

And when I think about my own inevitable decline, as I have begun to do, I sometimes see myself facing an existence absent any close human support.

And that is not an appealing prospect.

Carol appears to have fallen asleep. I will close this writing session. Clearly, there is more to think about this issue and will pick it up again when the time seems right.

A cold and very blustery early December day. Hardly any sun, constant howl of the wind, which has blown all remaining fallen leaves into the woods, leaving the browning grass exposed. Altogether it is a day ripe for dark thoughts.

I have come to the startlingly obvious realization that at least for me it is harder to be alone in the winter than the summer. When the weather outside is so inhospitable, from my point of view, the temptation is to burrow into the warmth both physical and emotional of one's house.

Now with the storm doors reinstalled and the gas burner recently checked and tuned up, my house is quite warm enough in the physical sense.

However, its emotional thermometer is dipping. Carol's body, in sleep, on the couch nudges that emotional temperature up a bit. But as I dried from my daily shower and noticed, as I do every day, Carol's towel hanging unused in its accustomed place next to mine, I experience a strong pang of loneliness, reminding me yet again that only I now use that bathroom.

The season is not the cause of this self-pitying mood; it is the amplifier.

And what it amplifies are the two realities within which I live. One is the patterns and artifacts of all the pre-disease years with Carol. The other is those same patterns and artifacts now forced into the present reality of the diminished Carol.

The link between the two is her physical presence. In recent days I have come to understand how important that is for me. It enables me to live a kind of lie, that the past reality of our lives together somehow continues into, and perhaps merges with, the present.

I call that a lie because intellectually I know it is false. Whatever we are experiencing now is its own new reality leading us toward a looming future of immeasurable difficulty. To forestall that future's arrival is reason to subscribe to the lie.

It's a maddeningly ambiguous place to be. I take her hand and squeeze. She tightens her grip as well. What exactly does that mean? Is it just an automatic muscle-to-muscle response, having nothing to do with her brain? In other words, is it just a response to stimulus, a neuron signal up to that portion of her brain that responds much as it does when you pull your hand away from something hot? Or on a level up, does it trigger a memory-based response, recalling the thousands of times her hand felt such pressure and responded to it? And if it does do that, does her brain connect that memory to me as the party of the second part? And even if it does so, which Steve is it responding to: the one actually holding her hand, or the one stored in her long-term memory?

About a week ago, there was a brief incident that shines a bright light on what I am trying to describe.

"You look pretty good," she had said.

A remark these days so totally unexpected. It echoed, sort of, in my memory as something she might have said once upon a time.

But now?

Take the sentence apart.

First, the "you." Is that me now or me in her memory?

That question is hugely important. We will come back to it.

Then what follows, "look pretty good."

There is no getting around the idea of physical attractiveness.

I had just come into the living room from the kitchen where I was starting to prepare supper. I had heard her call my name. Usually, when she does that, I find that she does not have a specific request or question or need. I ask her, and she sometimes says she has forgotten, or looks perplexed as to why I am even there.

This time was different. At least, her remark seems to suggest something else although what that might be, I have no idea. I came into the room. She looked at me, and said, "You look pretty good."

Not in a surprised way as though it was unexpected that I might look good. More of an appreciative way.

It is tempting to read too much into those four words.

Of course, I want to think that she is looking at me as her present-day husband. After all, those four words followed her calling my name. What other conclusion can I draw?

Well, for starters, there may be no connection between her summons and her observation.

Perhaps it is just like the light reaching us from a distant but now dead star. The light is still bright, but the source is no longer there.

Because of that ambiguity, I am, in a strange kind of way, comforted by Carol's quite noisy sleeping. She lies on her back, often breathing through an open mouth, producing a cacophony of snores and snorts that demand to be heard.

And I am happy to hear them.

Because they announce that she is still here in our mutual present, whatever shape that has.

Sometimes she murmurs unintelligibly. I imagine she is giving voice to her own struggle with these realities.

When those sounds stop, when she goes into a quiet sleep, that looming future presses itself into my consciousness with unrelenting force.

I wait for her to again call my name.

No Fig Leaf

A snowy afternoon. Doesn't look like serious accumulation yet. Glad I installed a new spark plug in the snowblower, which responded by starting up in a test run.

Carol sleeping in a half sitting up position with a weighted vest on her chest, as per the instructions of the physical therapist, who along with the occupational therapist, will be here shortly to continue their efforts to get Carol comfortable standing up. The vest places weight on the shoulders. The theory is that the pressure will increase the message sent by the neurons in the shoulder to the brain, thus increasing the brain's awareness of the body's position. This strategy was, in fact, suggested by Carol's first occupational therapist. At that time, Carol was still mobile, and we never took up the idea. I can only hope that this neuron stimulation will be strong to lessen Carol's fear of falling enough to permit her to stand, and perhaps even walk.

Therapists have arrived.

It is Friday night, two days later, and my mood darkens as it does at the beginning of every weekend when I know I will lack much human contact. It is approaching midnight and I just finished tomorrow's Times *crossword puzzle, perhaps delaying what I think I will be writing about, today's startling juxtaposition of the ordinary and the extraordinary. The ordinary included the second day of having to snow blow the driveway. The extraordinary is dealing with what happened two days ago when Carol had a seizure.*

The physical and occupational therapists were pushing Carol hard, as they had done in the past. But this time, things did not go well. As in their one fairly successful session a couple of weeks ago before an insurance issue interrupted their efforts, they managed to get Carol on her feet, into the transport chair, and on her feet again in the bathroom where they encouraged her to look at her own face in the mirror.

So far so good. I was in the living room, keeping my distance as I usually do so they can work without my looking over their shoulders. I heard what was going on. Carol was being congratulated for standing so well.

But then, she wasn't. They were going to change her nightgown. She seems to have become uncomfortable and resisted. Her voice rose. They decided to just get her back into the chair and wheel her to the couch.

They stopped next to the couch. Carol was sitting in the chair with her head drooped. Drool dripped from her mouth and some other liquid from her nose. She did not respond when spoken to. I watched as they lifted her up and placed her on the couch.

After some minutes she seemed to come out of whatever it was. I called the practice and had the therapist describe the incident. I got back on the phone and asked when someone could come out to check Carol.

That turned out to be the next evening. In the interim Carol pretty much regained her normal state, having eaten her supper, gone to sleep, awakened, as usual, had her breakfast, and so forth.

The doctor who came listened to my description of what I had witnessed. He said he had not been briefed. Perhaps he just wanted to hear what I could tell him.

I told him that although I had only seen epileptic fits in movies or on television, that is what it looked like to me. He agreed in the sense that he said he was quite sure that she had had a seizure.

A seizure. What exactly is that, I asked.

The brain resetting itself, he replied.

Not a stroke?

No, he said, a stroke would leave the person with weakness on one side or the other.

Why now, I asked.

She's over **60**, he replied; people over **60** are vulnerable to these kinds of seizures.

Connected to the dementia?

Can't say.

Cause?

Possibly stress.

Now, two days later during which Carol is as she was before, I have both pushed the seizure aside so as to go on with the business of living while being perfectly aware I need to take it out, stretch it onto a table, and examine it.

Thus, the juxtaposition with which I started.

Ran out of steam last night, so I resume this Saturday afternoon with a heavy snow shower turning the air white. I am not going anywhere today, and I don't expect any visitors. I will not clear the driveway until tomorrow.

I have been thinking about the quasi-artificial deadline that has been shaping my thinking concerning my continuing to serve as Carol's caregiver in our house. Her seizure, if that is what it was, makes that topic timely.

Months ago, I believe in late spring, I consulted with an elder attorney at a time when the realization hit me that I had better explore my situation in more depth. I had a number of questions concerning such matters as an existing power of attorney document, but the big elephant in the room demanding attention be paid to it involved how I would afford the cost of placing Carol in a skilled nursing facility.

My lifelong habit in dealing with such issues is to check out the lay of the land, see what my choices are and will be, and having done that, place the problem into mental storage, until such time as I would actually have to decide on a course of action.

That was my mindset when I consulted the attorney. I was then nowhere near making the gut-turning decision of placing Carol into a facility. I had already put her name on a waiting list for the Pavilions, a highly recommended place in town that apparently has a year waiting list. Doing that and gathering other relevant information was all I intended to do as a result of my consultation with the attorney.

We had gone over various matters but focused on the money issue. That turned out to provide additional support for my usual practice. Specifically, it alerted me to a date in the future at which the financial picture would change dramatically.

That date corresponded to the point when Carol would go on Medicare. Once on Medicare, she would become eligible for Medicaid support for a nursing facility, support sufficient to make that option affordable. My financial advisor had joined me at this meeting, so the attorney had been fully briefed on my resources. With that information, she offered an educated guess as to what my out-of-pocket costs might be, and they were such as to be affordable.

The attorney's advice some six or so months ago was to not do anything—she said to hang in—until Medicaid support was available.

That, of course, suited me just fine. It strengthened my resolve to keep Carol with me at home, if for no other reason than financial stability. It kind of took the decision out of my hands. Even if on certain days when freeing myself from my caregiving responsibilities seemed attractive, I could always tell myself, just wait, don't do anything precipitous.

I knew then that this reasoning was something of a diversion. In the first place, I realized that, if absolutely necessary, I could absorb the cost of a facility for the months leading to Medicaid coverage. The attorney had said she might be able to secure that coverage earlier, but it would be difficult.

In the second, and more important, way, it made the real

issue secondary, when I knew, if I wanted to be honest with myself, that it was, and is, primary.

And that is whatever the money parameters, the real decision resides in my heart. At what point, under what circumstances, or stress, or emotional exhaustion, will I be ready to leave behind the fiction of living with the Carol *that was,* and accept the reality that the Carol *that is* must be put into professional hands, and my doing that will in a very profound way change my life, knowing, as I do, that the change might be of minor concern to Carol herself. Someone else would attend to her, as I do now, and she might not remember from time to time who that person is, as she does not always seem to be aware of who I am.

That last, of course, is the hardest morsel to swallow, anticipating, perhaps, the possibility that when I would make my visits to her, she would not know who I was.

Until now, I did not realize just how devastating that would be, how difficult to accept the reality that from her perspective I no longer existed although her memory of me might linger indefinitely.

Carol is now within weeks of being Medicaid eligible.

I will have to confront my decision-making without the cover of needing to wait.

That is how it should be. Such a decision should be made in all of its hideous nakedness. No fig leafs. No diversions.

Just what it is on its own unforgiving terms.

In that regard, the image of her sitting almost lifeless in that chair stays with me. It is not so much the drool, or the mucus, if that is what it was, dripping from her nose. No, it was the way her head drooped as though never again would she lift it up, that and the failure to respond to words, a touch, or a squeeze of her hand.

I suppose in my mind at that moment it was like touching a corpse.

A hideous exaggeration of the facts, to be sure, but since when do emotions pay much attention to facts?

I saw in her inert being the time when she would no longer be, when all traces of the Carol that was would be irretrievably gone.

And, in a sense, that is not so wild an overreaction.

For her dementia has already put her on that train, which might, any day, leave the station.

Of Whiteness and Annihilation

Wind howling outside confirming winter weather advisory of snow starting tonight and continuing all day tomorrow with predicted accumulation perhaps a foot or more. That will most definitely complicate my schedule this week.

We will see. Such dire predictions have been wrong before. The wind rattling the window behind me, however, says not this time.

It's been five days since Carol's seizure, and there is no sign of a recurrence. If anything, her appetite seems better, not that appetite has anything to do with the seizure. The point is she seems very much like she was before. Even now, as our old mantle clock struck eleven o'clock, she yelled at it to shut up. Which is what she generally does.

I was about to say she was back to normal but had to correct myself because that word has lost any semblance of its usual meaning. What exactly does *normal* mean when applied to someone with dementia?

I'm sure I don't know.

What I can say is that her behavior, whatever word is used to describe it, does follow certain patterns and remains within the parameters thereby created. In that respect, she is back where she was before the seizure.

But this little exploration of semantics, so natural to me, raises difficult questions. If I can't define normalcy in the context of dementia, I also recognize that I try very hard to convince myself that a measure of the ordinary understanding of that word persists.

I am not exactly lying to myself. I know that much of what I do as caregiver, starting with hand-feeding her breakfast to settling her down on the couch for sleep, and everything in between, is anything but normal.

Still, I hang on to the slivers of behavior that enable me to, for a moment or two, buy the fiction that things are normal. From time to time, we do have snippets of conversation. Tonight, she asked me who Ed was. I replied that maybe she was thinking of her father's friend of that name. Yes, she said.

Did she actually remember Mr. Ed Brown who has been, I believe, gone for some time?

Perhaps.

When I told her about the snowstorm on its way, she nodded, a nonverbal affirmation that she knows all about the winters here.

Over the course of any day, there are not many of these moments. They tend to be overshadowed, or overwhelmed, by utterances and occasional behaviors formed by her dementia.

But when they do come, they are both precious and dangerous.

Precious because they lift my spirits, push off for a while the black cloud that hovers over us.

But dangerous precisely because that cloud is the new normal, however we want to define that term.

Once again in my chair across from Carol just falling asleep on the couch. For some reason she was in a combative mood, perhaps because she had been bathed by the aide and she does not like being so handled.

The major snowstorm did not materialize, and the winds have died down. Winter is settling in.

Tonight is the first night of Hanukkah. In years past, Carol would watch while I read the prayers and lit the menorah. She always encouraged me to maintain my hold on my Judaism. She bought me a three-volume history of Jews in New York and was happy to help prepare a Passover meal that we hosted for our close friends.

But this year there seemed no point to pull out the menorah and order the necessary candles online. For whom would I be doing this? The dog? Myself? The solitary nature of the activity just didn't make any sense to me.

Doctor just arrived to check Carol. I continue to be thankful for this new practice that offers home visits. Carol checks out fine physically, heart, bowels, blood pressure, pulse, all vitals good.

A medical professional confirms that Carol's physical self remains unchanged. Her mind, however, has not, and perhaps will not, find its stasis.

I attend to the former as best I can.

The only thing sure about the latter is that with slight up and down variations its own pronounced movement will be down.

Saturday night, an unusual writing time for me. But it has been a very quiet day, no more than a half dozen words exchanged with another person, in this case the window clerk at the local post office. The quiet is amplified by the unremitting white landscape. In "Desert Places," Robert Frost describes walking past a field being covered in snow, suggesting that the whiteness invites an apprehension of annihilation. One doesn't have to be literary to be somehow distraught gazing out of the window at a white blanket that covers all that is familiar with a blank stare coming back at you.

And so my antidote to such a feeling is to fill a white page on my laptop's screen with black words.

These weekends as I have no doubt said before are difficult. I cling to Carol's presence as nonverbal as it is for the most part. Oh, we squeeze out a few words back and forth that leave the impression of a conversation, but I know I am fooling myself.

Deliberately.

Which I do regularly, leading to my decision today that I would try to begin a program that would lead to Carol regaining her ability to stand.

And then to walk.

I would ever so gently have her take my hands and permit me to help her sit up straight. Our very comfortable and yielding sofa encourages you to sink back into it. It does take a little effort to push yourself into an upright position from which you can then get up onto your feet.

Of course, it did not work. At first, she seemed willing. But when I held out my hands, her fear won out and she just settled back into her usual half-reclining position.

I will try another day.

I do not want to give up just yet.

Perhaps I am motivated at this time by my shiny new leased Camry in our garage, the possession of which reinforces the idea that in some ways, life can move on in a positive direction. Carol loved cars and took exquisite care of her Subaru. I know she will never sit in that new car, never enjoy with me its comfort and power. That is beyond reasonable expectation. But if she were to get back on her feet, perhaps she would be able to get to a window where she could see it. That would be something.

Or maybe I am thinking of our daughter's visit next week and would like her to be able to see her mother standing up.

These are, in some ways, ridiculous motivations. But they are also quite real.

I know this disease is irreversible.

And yet I try.

A couple of days ago, I brought up from the basement the miniature Christmas tree we have had for years and years. It has a string of blue lights on it, some beads wrapped around it, and a handful of ornaments, including one that has our daughter's name on it, dated 1998. I plugged it in and got Carol looking in that right direction.

I convinced myself that she saw it and acknowledged its presence.

Maybe she actually did.

Looking back over what I have just written, a thought strikes me.

The white I began with is Carol's disease, covering what she was; no, covering is not a strong enough word, better to say obliterating day by day who she was. But even under this blanket of snow, as the stubble in Frost's poem still pokes through the white, are the shapes being covered, so the snow mimics those forms, there a rise indicating a chair on the deck, there a bulge where the watering can I left still sits.

It is those shapes and forms and no longer the things themselves that are like the traces of Carol still pushing through the obscuring, the suffocating, white of her disease.

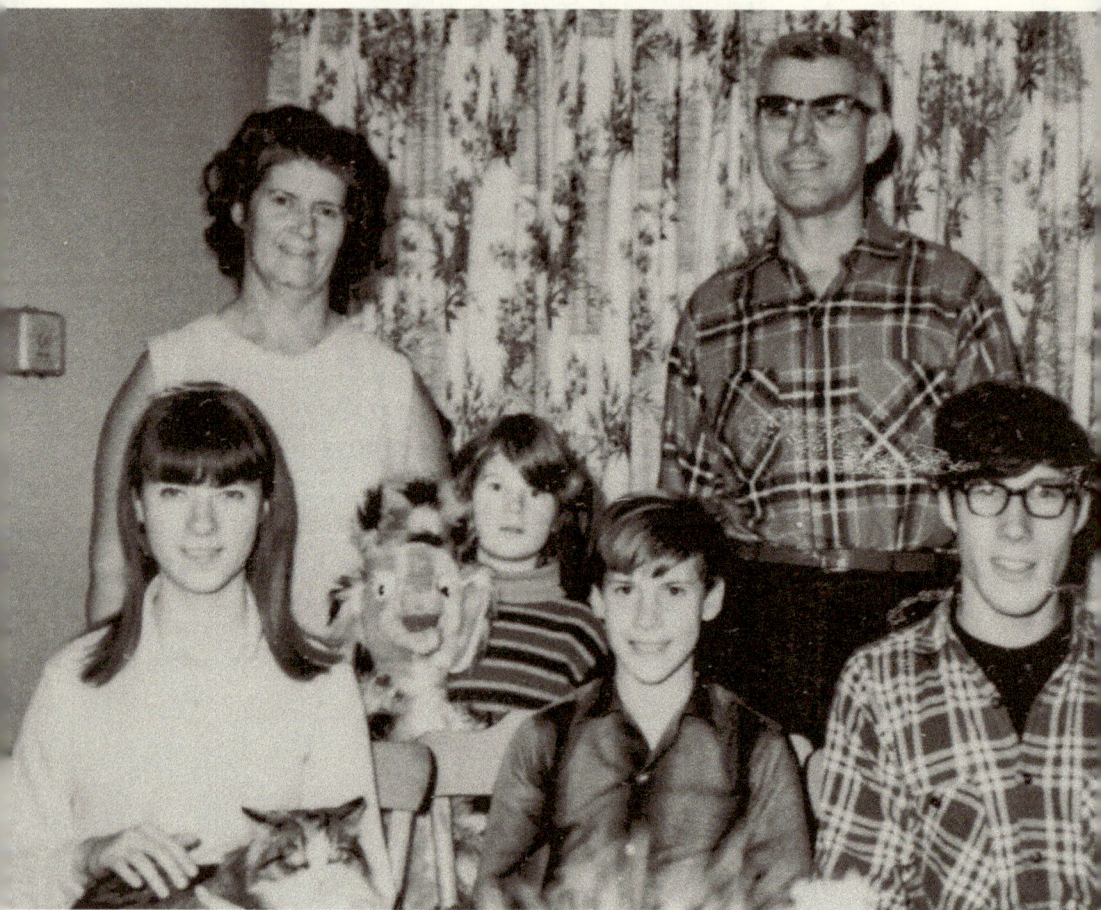

The Johnson family, ca. late 60s.
Top from left: Mary Johnson, Walter Johnson
Bottom from left: Carol, Jane, Ward, Dean

Holidays

Monday night. Carol asleep on the sofa. Dog in her bed.

Our daughter will be here Wednesday evening for a few days right before Christmas although she can't stay for the holiday, having to drive back in time to return to her job. I have tried to prepare her for what she will encounter, but there really is no way to do that.

Carol is oblivious to the holiday season, but she is sure that she has cancer. I cannot disabuse her of this notion.

That is not surprising. It is impossible to prove a negative. Even if she were thoroughly tested now, another mammogram, colonoscopy, administer any and all cancer screening tests and have all of them come back negative. That would not persuade someone who did not want to be persuaded.

So, the question is why Carol wants to believe she has cancer.

And I think I might have figured out an answer.

She must know on some level she is not right, by which I mean, not her former self. Of course, that is abundantly clear to even the most casual observer. But that fact perhaps has also made its way through her cognitive impairment.

She sees other people, primarily me and the caregiver relief aides, doing things she cannot any longer do. That much is a fact. And maybe even in some inchoate form a memory stirs in her head that once upon a time she did the same things, stood up by herself, fed herself, walked about the house.

That is the beginning of my hypothesis as to why she is so insistent in believing that she has cancer.

The next step in my developing guess is that she is angry.

Very angry.

Not all the time. Her mood is generally accepting of her condition.

But underneath that placid surface there might be seething anger. I've seen that anger erupt in profane expressions, usually when she is drowsing. Sometimes when she is fully asleep, she will start up and curse a presence her brain has manufactured.

So there is anger directed at a particular stimulus, one created by her mind. But perhaps there is also a discontent to which she cannot put a name, but which nonetheless nags at her sense of well-being to the point that she must respond to it.

So cancer jumps to mind. It is convenient. She did have cancer and was never the same after the treatment that got rid of it.

I'll go a step further. It is possible that she sees the cause/effect that is so clear to me. The cause of cancer, the effect of dementia.

At first glance, that causal relationship seems false. Of course, the cancer did not *cause* her dementia.

But the chemo no doubt accelerated it to a significant degree.

Carol is not making such a nuanced distinction.

She was high functioning before the cancer.

She is barely functional now.

She is angry and needs a target.

Cancer it is.

Christmas Eve and all is very, very quiet. Carol still up, the dog not yet in her bed, and I in my usual late-night chair. For some reason, I have found a station streaming unobtrusive classical music and I am listening with earbuds plugged into my laptop. I have always been an avid listener of music, often when I am working on the computer. I recall that when I was writing my dissertation decades ago, I had a radio on my desk tuned to WPAT from Paterson, New Jersey, which played easy listening music.

This holiday season is happening as though on another planet. I did not send out cards, in and of itself not so unusual as many people have abandoned that practice, switching to social media instead. We received a few cards, and I did bring up our miniature artificial tree with its string of blue lights. That, of course, was for Carol's benefit, as left to my own devices I would have left it in the basement. It is a relic from another time, a reminder of when we would be immersed into Carol's family's celebration, everyone gathering in her parents' house on Christmas Day. Carol shared her family's enthusiasm for the holiday, and so when our daughter was young in New York, we would have a full-sized tree, sometimes real, sometimes artificial, and once we moved here, I strung lights on this house.

Carol's family no longer gathers, as each nuclear family now goes its own way, a kind of natural evolution, I suppose.

But they are all celebrating.

We are not.

I told Carol a little while ago that it is Christmas Eve. She did not offer much of a response.

Not surprising.

Our daughter is now halfway back to Minnesota after a three-day visit. She will be completing her journey on Christmas Day.

For Carol and me, tomorrow will unfold as does every other day.

Putting all this together produces an eerie feeling of being on an isolated island in the midst of an ocean of unrestrained exuberance.

It is not terrible, just strange.

I can't decide how I feel about this.

I regret that Carol no longer can enjoy that celebratory holiday energy. But I don't really miss it. I was never fully part of it anyway.

Still, the feeling of being isolated, of dealing with Carol's dementia primarily by myself, is amplified by our detachment from the holiday festivities.

A week from now New Year's Eve will replicate this experience, perhaps with even more emphasis.

It was lovely having our daughter here for her brief visit. For those days, which included a dinner out with Carol's brother and wife, and Carol's sister, with the nephew staying with Carol, there was a whiff of normalcy.

Now that is gone up the chimney, down which will come no chubby little elf.

Late night after a fierce winter day, lots of snow, wind chills below zero, whiteouts that obscure the roads. I cleared the driveway to provide room for Tuesday's aide, but then watched the snow continue. Luckily, neighbor Rocco came by with his rider snowblower and a few more passes with that machine got the driveway clear again. Took my time going to town for groceries.

Yesterday's Christmas Day was absolutely quiet. The phone did not ring once, and that simply does not happen during this time of constant barrage of telemarketers and robocallers pitching Medicare Advantage plans.

I wished Carol a merry Christmas. She kind of smiled, but I am not sure what to make of the response. I've pointed out our little fake Christmas tree and told her which cards had come. In that regard, she responds to the names, it seems, much more fully than the holiday itself. Today, a card came from Etta, one of her very old friends from the time she was working in New York. Etta's name registered strongly and elicited a clear and loud repetition. I seem to remember that I took dictation from Carol for a letter to Etta some time ago when Carol's head was still good, but her handwriting had failed her.

Another card came from Jeff, my office mate for my last year's teaching. Carol also responded to his name, but actually more to my recalling that Jeff's wife Sue is a judge. From time to time, Carol still reminds me that she is a lawyer.

After that long quiet Christmas Day I was in a funny mood,

one that is hard to describe. I wasn't down, nor was I up. But I surely lacked any ambition or inspiration to do anything, which is unusual for me. From ten o'clock on, most evenings, my energy revs up, and I find something to do, write, read, or watch the news or a sports event if one of my teams happens to be on.

But not last night. I sat in the TV room looking for something to watch. It was way too early for me to consider sleep. Carol called me in as she sometimes does after she has gone to sleep herself. This time, she appeared to be upset about something, but she could not tell me what.

I sat with her, holding her hands for a good while until she settled back to sleep. Occasions like that encourage me to continue with our present arrangements.

I still was neither sleepy nor motivated to do anything.

I opted for mindless entertainment and watched the latest Jason Bourne movie.

It was peculiarly satisfying to let Hollywood take hold of my mind and chase everything else away.

A fitting end to our non-celebratory holiday, the sensory overload emanating from the TV screen, the obliterating white from the snowstorm outside, both in their very different ways providing analgesic relief, a couple of hours during which I thought about nothing.

These days nothing is sometimes better than the somethings I have to think about.

New Year's Eve

A couple of days after Christmas, snowed in, unremitting boredom only interrupted by the daily war against the drifts on the driveway—thank you persistent northerly winds—and the resumption of calls from telemarketers on behalf of insurance companies peddling add-ons to Medicare coverage. One such call came in today with a local number and just the beginning of our town's name on the caller ID. Thinking it might be some entity I actually had a connection to, I picked up the line only to be confronted with a woman clearly reading a pitch from a script, who would not, could not, stop long enough to answer a simple question as to the purpose of the call. I imagine some college student trying to earn a few bucks over semester break. I could have been kinder, let her finish her pitch, but I had just come in from doing the driveway and could not yet feel my fingers, and so I hung up.

For variety, just received a call from the political party I support.

From day to day, there is little change in Carol's condition. Her appetite, if anything, seems stronger. Her mood is occasionally combative but not more so than before, and perhaps a little less. She is taking her meds more readily. Maybe it helps that I have taken to accompanying the dispensing of pills by counting in Spanish, German, or French—I can usually get up to six or seven in each—or by reciting the old rhyme that starts "One, two, buckle my shoe," as I feed her the pill.

Because of this seeming stability and encouraged by a couple of indications of a willingness to get onto her feet, I decided to try to maneuver her into the transport chair to eat with us while our daughter was here, and we were joined by our nephew. I thought I could lift her up while he stopped the chair from sliding on our slick wooden floor.

The first part sort of went okay. I wrapped my arms around her and lifted her up, then lowered her onto the chair. However, she was complaining mightily the whole time, in an absolute panic, and slid off the seat before we had a chance to secure her with the seat belt.

I will not try again.

If we get another physical therapist in after the new year when she is on Medicare so that insurance will not again be an issue, I'll consider another attempt.

Apparently, although I know Carol's disabilities are not reversible, I cling to the possibility that there may be effective compensation strategies.

I have always been stubborn in pursuit of certain goals.

So be it in this case.

I will know that we did not go down without a fight.

In the library the Friday before New Year's Eve on Sunday. No other patrons, just a staff member shelving books. Caregiver relief aide will be with Carol for a little more than another hour, and I am back from town getting a small repair done on my glasses. Besides my laptop I've brought in the manual for the navigation and multimedia systems of my new Camry, a substantial tome. Apparently, these systems can do marvelous things, including responding to voice prompts. There's a bit of a learning curve involved, but I don't mind.

This morning Carol awoke sobbing, something about her mother. The best I could make out was she was unhappy that she could not either go to, or see, her mother. I considered reminding her that her mother was in the nursing home but chose instead to just hold her hand until she quieted down, which she did after a short while. I then said it was time for breakfast, and she seemed content with that.

This incident reminded me of episodes early in the onset of

her disease, where she would awaken convinced that somebody had died. I did not at that time understand that these events were a product of her dementia. I knew something wasn't right, but I could not put a name to whatever it was.

I now imagine they were some sort of hallucination. She would say that the information came to her through the air waves. My response, uninformed as it then was, was that had somebody died we would have heard through the more usual method of a telephone call. The telephone hadn't rung; hence, nobody had died.

Needless to say, she was not always convinced of this logic although through repetition the response did gain some traction with her. I do recall, however, one time when nothing would dislodge the fixed idea in her head that her cousin in Virginia had died, not only that he was now deceased, but he was so as the result of an accident while he was driving, I believe, a truck.

Perhaps now, I would just let that idea go, but then I tried to correct it, going so far as calling the last number we had for him—we were not in especially close contact with this individual—and spoke with someone, I don't recall who, from whom we learned that although he had moved he was above ground and quite well.

Over time, several other family members' deaths occurred to her, and I would repeat the mantra, no phone call, nobody is dead, and that worked.

There have been no such incidents for quite some time, and I don't think the one this morning was of that kind. Quite what it was, I still do not understand. I am aware that sometimes Carol will start laughing, as though someone has just told her a joke. When I once asked who it was, she answered, it was herself. She never was much of a joke teller, but I'd rather she be doing that than sobbing.

New Year's Eve. Carol asleep on the couch after a late dinner. The dog asleep on the floor near the chair on which I am sitting. I checked the TV for something to watch, including shows and movies I had recorded. Nothing interested me.

We've had serious snow the past few days, probably a couple of feet although I haven't heard an official determination. I managed to get out to the store this morning as part of my Sunday routine, New York Times *for me, a muffin for Carol.*

It somehow seems fitting that the weather should add to my feelings of isolation this festive season.

I am somehow reminded of a New Year's Eve some sixty or more years ago. I do not know why this one sticks in my mind, nor why it intrudes into my consciousness tonight.

But it does, so I'll take a look at it.

I was probably about twelve, maybe a little older. We had moved from the two-family house where we were the tenants on the second floor. The move was sudden—a dispute with the landlord. I don't know now, nor did I know then, the particulars. What I do know is that we moved in the middle of the school year when I was in the sixth grade. Another upstairs apartment some twenty-eight blocks west on the very same Avenue I.

I am not sure if my sister was still living with us. She got married when I was thirteen or fourteen. In any case, she would not have been home on New Year's Eve.

Nor my parents that year although I don't recall their going out much on holidays.

Thus, I was home alone, too young to go out to my own party, or perhaps too new to the neighborhood if there were any celebrants of my age I could have joined.

I don't remember what I did that night. I am quite sure I did not watch television. I don't know what would have been on then in the middle to late fifties.

The only detail that, weirdly, is fixed in my memory is a calendar given out by the Chinese restaurant on Avenue J. I can recall what it looked like. Each page was a week, with several lines for each day where notes could be written. It was probably about eight to ten inches high and maybe six or seven inches wide with a dark brown back. The name of the restaurant was somewhere, either on the backing above the pages, or perhaps on each page. I do not remember which.

It makes some sense that I would associate this calendar with New Year's Eve. It would have been brand spanking new for the new year.

But that is all I recall of that evening.

I try to recapture my mood. Words like weird, detached, and alienated come to mind. Not quite lonely although that would seem natural in a situation in which my own family was out somewhere celebrating.

Nor can I say that I felt angry.

Perhaps the best word is estranged. In my own little non-celebratory bunker.

Which is exactly how I feel tonight.

I told Carol it was New Year's Eve. I am not sure that meant anything much to her. She never had a head for time. I'm sure it was a struggle for her to keep to necessary school and work schedules. But she surely did do that right through jobs, university, and law school.

Without that imposed structure she had great difficulty. She had to write things down, usually in a yearly planner. When I went out for a bike ride, she would record the time I left.

It struck me as painfully inappropriate—best word I can come up with—that the other day we received in the mail quite a lovely, good-sized, faux leather-bound planner from our financial advisers.

Just the kind of thing Carol would have loved.

I have a calendar on my phone synced to my computer.

But Carol never moved comfortably into the digital world. This planner would have suited her perhaps as recently as a year ago.

But not now.

Not now when one day blends into another for her, as do the weeks, and the months.

And the years.

So, perhaps I will awaken her at midnight.

Or maybe not.

Let her sleep. The new year is pretty much irrelevant.

To both of us.

Coda: Tuned to streaming WQXR from NYC, which was offering New Year's special of classical music's greatest hits and listened to the end of Beethoven's 7th and all of his 9th. The station let the music play right through midnight so that instead of watching the ball drop, my earbuds were filled with the glorious "Ode to Joy."

Perfect.

Time is irrelevant listening to timeless music.

When the music ended, I succumbed, acknowledged the present moment, and nudged Carol awake and wished her a happy new year.

She smiled in recognition and went back to sleep.

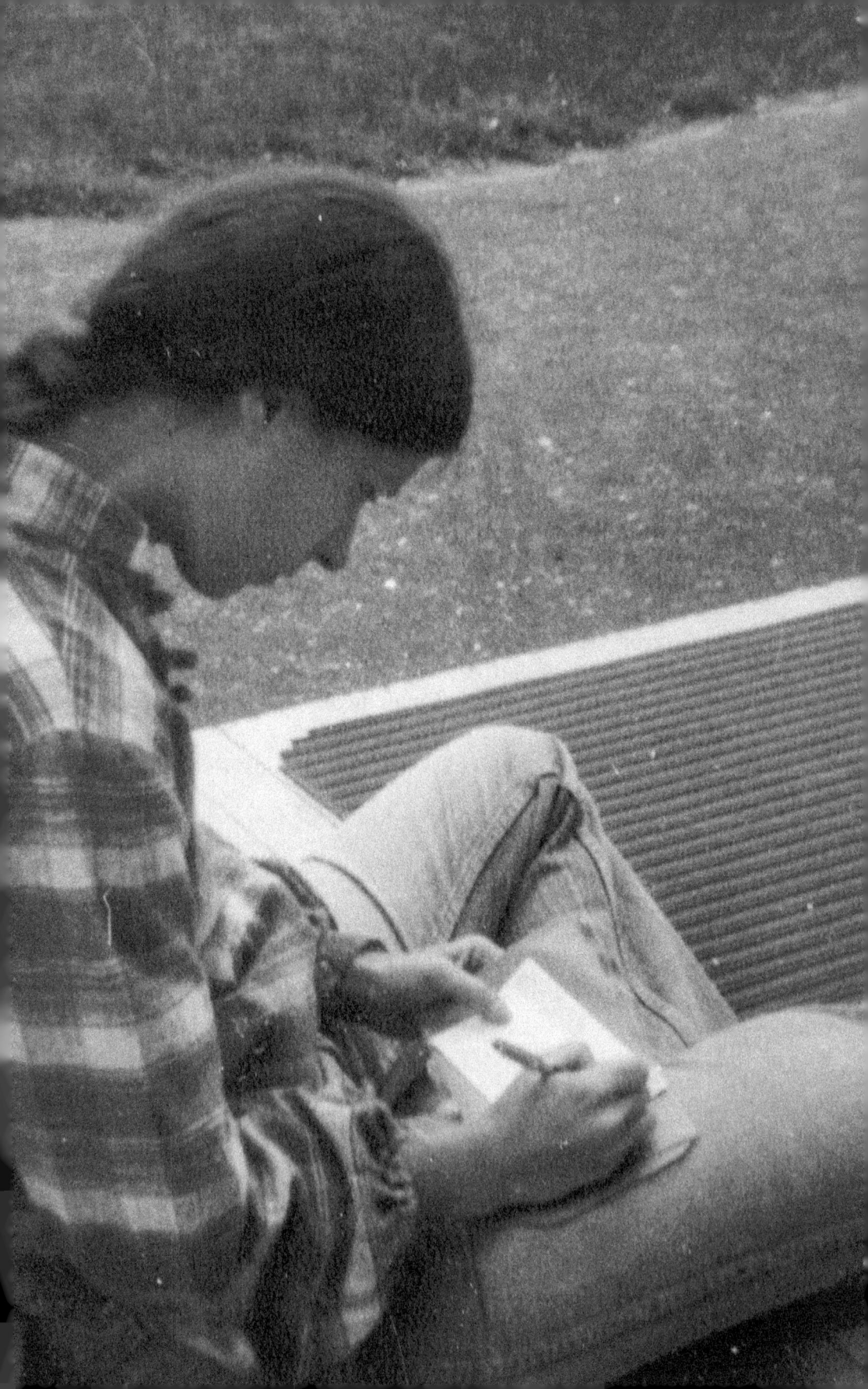

Two Writers and a Deity Named George

Caregiver relief aide is here. I am up in my office not caring to deal with cold and snow to go someplace else. The dog is confused. Decided to stay downstairs. Not sure if I should feel slighted.

Yesterday, I received an envelope containing three author copies of *Rosebud*, a nationally circulated literary magazine in which appears my short story "Mumblety-peg," first written as one of a series of linked stories in 1979. The idea was to produce a kind of fake novel and publish it as a book. That never happened. But over the years I revisited the individual stories, revised them, and sought publication, a process that has been largely successful.

This story is one of the last to find a home. Interestingly, it is the one that came closest to being a huge success as it made its way up the slush pile (heaps of unsolicited submissions) of the *Atlantic* all the way to the desk of the esteemed fiction editor C. Michael Curtis who sent me a handwritten rejection note, saying only the story was too dark for him.

I mention all of this as preface to the sad fact that I cannot really share this late coming good news with Carol. I, of course, mentioned it. Held up the magazine in front of her eyes and received the slightest hint of a response.

Had Carol not been much involved in my writing career, her disease-caused indifference at this time would not strike such a sour note. But just the opposite is the case. If we didn't originally get together through writing, writing surely was a shared passion, and we were intimately involved in each other's careers. Mine was further along because I am ten years older and had started sooner.

<<< Carol at her favorite activity, writing by hand.

But she quickly established her own standing as a fine and award-winning short story writer. To the immediate point, however, she was also an excellent editor and gave all of my work the most thorough going over, complete with marginal notes in her beautiful hand. Naturally, I didn't always agree, but that is any writer's privilege, and she would return the favor when I made suggestions concerning her work.

All that, of course, is now lost.

When her disease hit her, she was trying to market her stories as a collection as well as conquer the challenges of a novel.

I had just finished writing a new novel. At that time, she could no longer provide editorial response, but she was an active cheerleader.

That, too, is gone.

We were very different writers in many ways. In part that was the case because our backgrounds were so dissimilar, I from an urban environment, she having grown up on a farm. And of course, gender probably contributed to the differences as well. She was far more visual than I while I probably concentrated a bit more on plot. Our methods contrasted as well. She had to have long stretches away from all distraction while I was very used to working in short snatches, much as I am doing now.

We respected each other's approach to writing and, for the most part, did not try to impose our ways or interests on the other. Although, when asked for an opinion, we offered what each thought was the best from our own perspective.

We had separate personal libraries. When we had floor-to-ceiling bookcases installed in the dining room on the wall that led through a doorway to the kitchen, we each took half. We didn't discuss that decision because it was perfectly natural. We simply did not read the same kinds of books. In fact, I don't think I can recall more than a handful of instances, if that many, when one of us would pick up a book that the other had enjoyed.

We did read each other's work and tried to put on a critic's hat and ignore the inevitable intrusion of emotions arising from our relationship as husband and wife. That was not always an easy path to walk.

For both of us.

In looking through her journal that I found in her out building office a while ago, I saw a couple of places where she expressed her sensitivity to the pressure she perceived came from me to work as a writer more as I do.

Still I think we managed it quite well. Our respective talents made that a bit easier.

The receipt of my author copies brings back all of this, our shared passion for writing and support for each other's work.

It creates a void for me that will not be filled.

Late on a Thursday night of a day that was mostly okay, especially in terms of the weather. After a stretch of arctic cold and accumulating snow, the temperature rose to fifty. We are promised, however, that winter will return.

Carol is asleep on the couch, occasionally filling the air with a snorting kind of snore. I don't think it is indicative of a health issue, rather the product of sleeping on her back with her mouth half open.

Had lunch with my guys, three today, one usual attendee couldn't make it, but my neighbor, back from the Mayo Clinic in Minnesota where his wife is receiving stem cell therapy, rejoined us.

Although Carol has been eating with good appetite the past week or so, today she was not interested in the wrap I brought back for her, nor did she have much enthusiasm for supper. I will have to pay attention to her appetite. I recall hearing that dementia can diminish interest in food.

I don't have much energy, so I hope to pick this up tomorrow afternoon in the library.

Friday afternoon and unfortunately, the weather predictions for today were accurate. Temperature in the teens, strong north winds, rain into snow leaving ice everywhere. Arriving at the library, I see only one car. It's not a holiday, so school should be open. It turns out school was closed because of ice, and the one car belongs to a library clerk who chose to come despite the weather to get some of her work done. As I sit here, another employee comes in.

For the past couple of weeks, it is as if there's a god looking down at me and deciding that I don't have enough to do with being the caregiver for Carol. After all she does sleep a lot during the day.

So, this deity, I will call him George, for no particular reason except that appellation usually pops into my head when I try to come up with a name. I truly don't understand my connection to it. I believe I have only known one George my whole life, a fellow who was a colleague of mine on the college newspaper. I recall he got himself a gig reviewing restaurants for a local paper. He ate out often for free.

My imagined deity seems to have decided to give me things to do, dropping a turd into my life at regular intervals. Not a big lump, mind you, but a small one, say the kind you might carelessly step on.

Small, yes, but still you have to take the time to scrape it off your shoe, a tedious and unpleasant chore.

I won't bother with the details, just the topics. On various days, I have had to deal with my email shutting down, my Amazon account being compromised, both of these more than once, and then on one day the postal mail presenting me with two insurance billing problems, each one filling up a day's free time to deal with.

All of them like that squished turd on a shoe, not of great consequence, although the Amazon one with its possible credit card implications potentially rising to that level, but the others that while demanding to be confronted like the pungent residue on the shoe, fall into the category of ordinary life irritations.

And that, for me, and perversely, is their charm. I mention them to Carol who seems not to process anything more than the fact that I am bothered by something that her mind no longer relates to. I suppose I give voice to the issues for her attention out of long habit or perhaps an outdated sense of responsibility. She was, after all, my life partner, and I can kind of pretend she is still.

And speaking about these annoyances provides a little bit of release.

More important, though, is the fact that these problems are useful distractions. They give me something quite concrete to deal with. Better still, they can be resolved, ultimately, after battling through phone menus and individuals unable to help, until finally reaching the person with the competence and authority to do what is necessary to remove the problem.

And, thus, metaphorically, my shoe is once again clean.

The sudden January thaw has given me another such problem, but one I will deal with after the winter. The thaw released huge chunks of ice from our roof. One of these landed on the corner of the railing of our deck, smashing the wood.

It happens that corner had been hit the same way last winter, and the newly damaged part is the replacement piece installed last spring.

And who says George doesn't have a sense of humor. Or that he does not look ahead.

And, no, I will not try to explain why my imagined deity is male.

Carol, of course, is unaware of all this. The dog does sense my irritation and decides her bed is calling.

I don't think George has any plans for Carol.

That job has been taken by her disease, for which I did not have to invent a name.

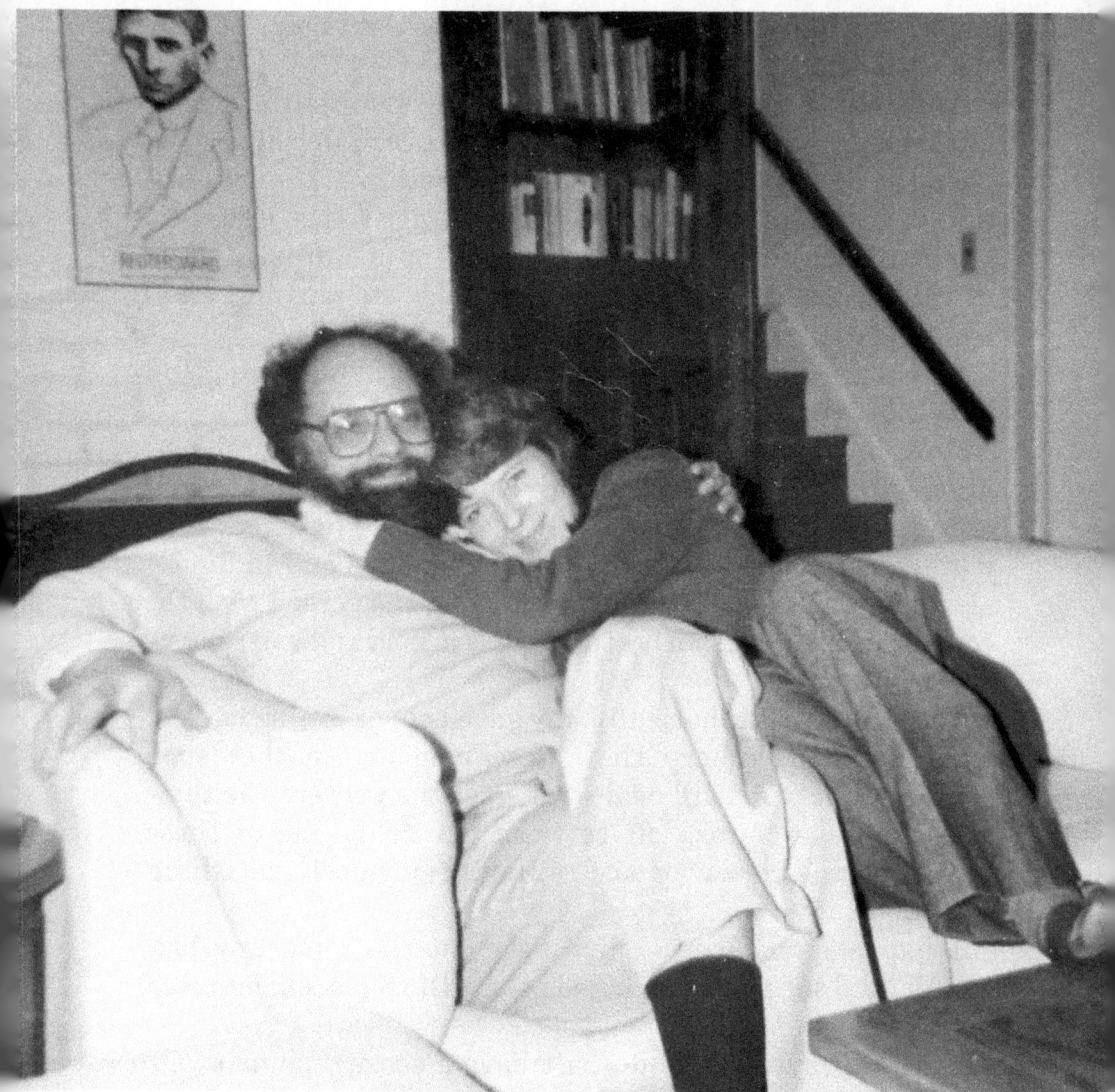

Between Past and Present

Near midnight on Sunday. Watched a two-hour season premiere of PBS's Victoria *alone, although the dog slept through the show, lying, as she usually does, on the floor in the TV room.*

I did think of inviting Carol to join me, as we always watched Masterpiece *together on Sunday nights. And she had a particular interest in Queen Victoria. One of the last books we got for her was the new, massive biography of the queen. When it was clear, however, that she could no longer process words on the page I read the book aloud to her until her attention flagged and she lost interest.*

So the combination of our past habit of watching this show together and her interest in Victoria *made me consider asking her to join me. A little reflection, though, convinced me to not even try. Getting her into the room would have been a formidable task, and then, even more important, I remembered that she could no longer focus on the visual stimuli offered by the television.*

This morning upon waking, Carol asked, "Steve, are you here?"

That brought a silly smile to my face. I was convinced she was aware that she was directing her question to the present me, not the remembered me.

I'm not sure why I was so sure. It was probably something in the tone of her voice. It had a certainty to it as though she was certain that I was nearby, the actual physical me, and not the shadowy me of memory.

This incident fits a recent pattern. For the while, her condition seems to have stabilized, including occasions of what appear to be a stronger connection to the present moment.

These moments remain scattered and outnumbered, to be sure, by the times when her mind seems elsewhere. In fact, today she was having persistent conversations with person or persons unknown. These appeared to be delightful interactions, accompanied by laughter.

But they clearly had nothing to do with me. Or the dog.

And herein is the horrible dilemma provided by this disease. The teasing, tantalizing moments that trap me into responding as though they indicate some kind of return to normalcy.

They do not so indicate.

I know that.

But I let myself be fooled each time anyway.

Again, late, and I'm tired. This Monday was Martin Luther King Jr. Day. No mail, few calls. I spent a fair amount of time setting up appointments for matters I have been ignoring, such as to the periodontist, or to the elder attorney with whom I want to explore the possibilities of Medicaid for Carol.

I'll scratch out what I can, continuing where I left off.

A day later and Carol woke up with an intensified fear of falling. I had to reassure her verbally several times, and then when those measures failed, I positioned myself lying down on the sofa so as to be able to hold her hand or stroke her cheek to reassure her that she was perfectly safe.

When this fear persisted even after breakfast, I realized I had not yet administered her morning meds. Perhaps that had something to do with the continuing problem. In any event, after a while she seemed to settle down without the fear.

This is the up and down that people talk about, the good day/bad day syndrome. I honestly don't know if the good days are worth the inevitable bad that follows. And to talk about days is a misnomer. The changes are not that regular, predictable, or evenly spaced out.

After this rough start, the day then moved to a kind of ordinary pattern during which I offered, and she accepted,

BLTs for lunch. She didn't sleep as much during the afternoon as she usually does, and then ate a good supper of salmon, rice, and yellow squash.

Later in the evening, I asked her if she wanted me to read one of her stories to her. I had put two journals containing her work on the table next to the sofa so that the aides could read to her. One had tried but told me that Carol had no interest. Nonetheless, I asked her tonight if she would like to hear her story, and she assented.

I read "Wings to Follow," all of it, and she listened attentively, smiling at lines she apparently remembered. I'm not sure when, or even if, I ever read the story, at least in its finished form. Reading it tonight reminded me, if I needed reminding, how good a writer Carol was. Simply put, this is a hell of a story. Two Native American sisters: one runs a bar, and the other is planning to travel, somehow, to the Upper Peninsula of Michigan to their mother's village.

It's all done so well, the simple plot, the relationship between the sisters, the characterizations, particularly of the older, bar-keeping sister, the language, and the ending. I am a student of endings because they are so hard to get right, and feel so good when they are, but so often do I see ones that simply do not satisfy. This story ends on a perfectly pitched note.

I am offering all of this, not as Carol's husband but wearing my writer/professor's hat.

A curious coincidence needs to be mentioned as well. At one point, the older sister mocks an arrogant teenager wielding a knife and uses the word "mumblety-peg."

The title of my just published story.

Which I am reasonably sure Carol never read because I wrote it before I met her.

If I believed in some mystical forces, this would be proof.

As she was getting ready for sleep, she said she was glad to have me.

That's as good as it is going to get.

I know that.

And it will not last
I know that as well.

But maybe the lesson here is simply to live in the moment, knowing that it offers no guidance to the next moment. That recognition, if I can hold onto it, will be a huge help.

After lunch the next day. I read a few pages to Carol from Love Medicine, *one of her favorite books, a section describing Grandfather's dementia which in some ways could be applied to Carol. He has little memory, and what memory he has is long-term, so he confuses the past with his present. There is one persuasive difference, however, between Erdrich's imagined picture of dementia and Carol's actual condition. Erdrich says Grandfather's loss of memory is a gain in that it enables him to forget things from his life he'd rather not remember. Carol, however, draws from the reservoir of her long-term memory things she likes to recall, such as that she was a lawyer. In fact, she doesn't use the past tense, she says she is a lawyer, and tonight she was talking about having to work.*

For the past couple of days, we seem to have returned to a version of the two Steves. This time it's a little more subtle or nuanced.

First it comes on the heels of a few occasions when Carol seemed very much in the present moment, such as when I was reading to her. During these occasions, I could easily permit myself to enjoy what is essentially a fiction or an illusion, that for those few minutes she was herself, and in being herself, she was fully aware of who I was.

But when I came home from an appointment in town yesterday, the aide said that Carol had been asking for me the whole time I was gone. And then last night, and again after breakfast this morning, she called my name literally every few minutes. I would respond, ask her what she wanted or needed.

She didn't say.

I would return to whatever I was doing, reading the paper or doing something on the computer, and again and again, every few minutes, she would call out for Steve. I stopped what I was doing, and went to sit next to her, take her hand, try to see what was going on in her head. When again she asked for Steve, I told her I was right there.

She seemed to accept that I was Steve. But I could not shake the idea that even though she acknowledged I was Steve, even though she indicated she understood that not only was I Steve, I was also the husband she was asking for, that in spite of these confirmations of who I was, she was still looking for some other Steve.

She would accept the present reality of me as Steve.

But in some way she was still conjuring up, and hoping to see, the Steve locked in her memory.

Her birthday is next week. I will get her roses. She will even in her confused state enjoy them.

But I am not sure she will know which Steve gave them to her.

I just have to live with that.

Of Living Room Ambiance
and a Box of Pictures

The weather has warmed for the while. It rained pretty much all day, and much of the snow is gone.

Carol is sleeping noisily on the couch with her mouth open.

A busy day of problem-solving punctuated by a visit from the nurse practitioner along with a student doing her practicum to check on the possibility, raised by one of the aides, that Carol has a urinary tract infection. They did not find any evidence of that.

With a fair degree of reluctance, I agreed to get a hospital bed for Carol. This is a huge step. I have been resisting for emotional, not practical, reasons, but practicality finally won out.

On the surface, my resistance was aesthetic. I did not want to change our living space into a medical facility. To be sure, there are medical devices scattered about: the travel chair near the steps reminding me of when Carol would ride in it, dismount, and climb to our bedroom, the cane in one corner, the two walkers in another corner, the grab bars in doorways and on walls leading to the steps, the shower bench and stool in Carol's office, all of these obvious indicators of our attempts to deal with the disease's progressively debilitating effects.

But in spite of them, somehow from my perspective they did not change the ambiance of our living space. They were like the dog's hair shed onto the floor, annoying but not visually offensive enough to change the character of the rooms in which they are stored.

The bed, though, is a different story. It will dominate the living room simply by virtue of its size. We might be using the sofas as our beds now, but they are still sofas. The hospital bed does not belong in our living room. The other items can be removed and stored, for they no longer serve their purpose. But the bed is its own purpose.

Like the sofa, the end table, and the cocktail table that provide the configuration of the living room, the bed is itself a piece of furniture. It belongs in a bedroom. Installed in our living room it imposes, it dominates, it demands its presence be recognized as signaling something profound.

Its presence states that we are crossing a line in our long journey away from the then toward a new now, one from which there is no turning back.

The misplaced bed, no doubt, will remain where it is until its occupant no longer needs it.

Another January teaser day, temperatures reaching toward fifty, the sun out, and graying snow melting. My head knows this is a mirage like the oasis in the desert of the winter, but as folks around here say, sure, but enjoy it.

In the library, back from a quick hop to town to buy a half dozen roses, three red, three white, for Carol's birthday. I declined the offer of a clip-on card on which to write a note. Since she can no longer read, I didn't see the point.

I placed the flowers on the lid of the wood stove I decided not to use this winter, as one thing too many. The foot of the hospital bed nudges the stove, so that the flowers will be in Carol's direct line of vision.

I directed her attention to them and was rewarded with an appreciative smile.

Last night as I came down the stairs after brushing my teeth, a title for a piece of writing jumped into my head: A Tale of Two Toothbrushes.

So here it is.

One toothbrush in the upstairs bathroom.

The other one in the downstairs bathroom.

Both are inexpensive battery driven models I bought some time ago, one for each of us. Mine is the one upstairs, Carol's the one downstairs, sitting next to her toothpaste on a shelf in that guest bathroom.

However, I have pretty much stopped trying to brush her teeth with her electric toothbrush. I have, instead, switched to disposable swabs. But the electric toothbrush remains in the downstairs bathroom, and sometimes I use it instead of mine upstairs. Each night when I am ready for sleep, I decide which toothbrush to use. If I am tired, I will opt for Carol's. There is no reason to worry about germs. Still, it feels a little odd because, as in so many other ways, using her toothbrush is an acceptance of the now. First because it is hers and she no longer uses it. And second because to employ that toothbrush I have to do so in the guest bathroom.

On the other hand, when I haul my weary carcass upstairs into the main bathroom and take my toothbrush and my toothpaste off my shelf in that bathroom, I am immersing myself into the then.

Today was Carol's birthday, and I was pleased that her sister Jane came by to wish her a happy one and to give her a card.

In all honesty, I don't think her birthday registered much in Carol's mind. She smiled at the flowers I bought for her, but thereafter did not seem to pay them much attention. Similarly, she responded only briefly when I showed her the few cards that arrived or relayed the digital best wishes from an old New York friend, a fellow Aquarian.

So tonight, after a day uneventful except for Jane's visit, and otherwise perfectly ordinary including my going to town for groceries, I am in my chair and Carol has fallen asleep.

This past weekend, Laura, our sister-in-law, brought a sizable, lidded plastic box containing photos that had been among Carol's family's material I had given some time ago to both Jane and Laura. In going through all of that stuff,

Laura had found a trove of photographs specifically relevant to us.

I took a brief look at the contents of the box, which I had set on the dining room table. The window in that room faces west, and as I looked up from the box and through that window, I noticed how the late afternoon sun emphasized the gray grime on the glass.

I know that grime would have irritated Carol.

One of the few things we disagreed about was the need to keep windows clean. As far as I can remember the windows in the apartments in Brooklyn I lived in both as a child, and as a young adult, were never washed and as a result always wore a layer of grime. If you wanted to see clearly, you'd open the window.

I have no idea how often the windows in Carol's house were cleaned. I do know that her heating engineer father had the windows of the house he had had built permanently sealed shut to keep out as much cold air as possible. How clear they were I do not know, so I cannot assume that their relative cleanness had anything to do with Carol's preference in this regard.

However, what I do know is that Carol was an intensely visual person. That point was driven home with considerable force by the sheer volume of the photographs in the box that Laura brought to me.

Of course, I always knew Carol loved photography. We have enlargements of some of her photos on the wall. And there are about half a dozen substantial photo albums on an otherwise empty bookcase in our basement apartment.

But what is now clear is that the albums represent a screening process that selected those shots worthy of being saved. What was in the box, however, was the raw material. I do not know if pictures of the same places and events are in those albums, so that the box material is the rejects.

I don't think so.

Because what's in the box, primarily, are the envelopes from that pre-digital age that came back from whatever developing service we were using, which provided two copies of every picture. And there were no single prints, suggesting that a picture had been removed and placed in the album, leaving its mate in the envelope. So I don't know why none of these pictures, which were shot between 1999 and 2000, as indicated not only by the obvious ages of the people, most easily established by those of our daughter, but also by the dates stamped on the envelopes, were put into an album.

I did not immediately dig into this material. I was apprehensive.

I would be immersing myself in our past, and I was not sure how ready I was so to do. But I began, tentatively, and then gained some confidence and moved through the envelopes with some pace.

As I flipped through the pictures, I found myself largely unable to identify locations other than the ones that clearly showed themselves to be our house and grounds on Long Island. The bulk of the others seemed to be from our various vacation trips, but try as I would, I could not remember where we went those two years. Since there were a lot of beach and water shots, I guessed Cape Cod. But not all the water pictures suggested oceanfront locales as there were ones showing Carol and Danielle in a canoe. Possibly that was from our trip to Isle Royale, and there were a couple that were taken from what appeared to be the seats in a boat such as the one we took across Lake Superior to that island.

Still others in a different part of the box were very obviously shot on our trip up to the Bread and Puppet summer festival in Glover, Vermont.

Or our drive out to South Dakota.

I realize as I tried to locate the where of these pictures, I was distracting myself from what I had feared.

That I would too forcefully be immersed in the then, and at our most relaxed and happiest times. We both loved to travel, particularly car trips.

Even when our vehicles were of questionable reliability

such as the aging Corolla that carried us up to Vermont for which the mountains were something of a challenge.

But then I realized something else.

Carol appeared in very few of the pictures.

Naturally enough. She was the photographer. Her subjects were our daughter, occasionally me, and predominantly whatever was interesting in the scenery, whether it was the buffalo herd in South Dakota, or the whale somewhere in the Atlantic, and in fact, water anywhere—she always loved water. One of the reasons we bought our present house is the distant view we have of the east arm of Grand Traverse Bay.

So for my first excursions into these pictures, I was spared the trauma of seeing more than a handful of images of Carol in the prime years of her young motherhood.

Later, as I dug further, I did come into another batch that was largely of her. I could not pin down the circumstances but there they were.

They hurt. But not as much as I thought they would. Even now, as I hear Carol's labored breathing in her sleep, reminding me of the now, I find myself somewhat better able to deal with the then.

I suppose that is some sort of progress.

Henry, William, and Rowing

Winter has returned after a brief hiatus. This morning after breakfast, I cleared five or six inches of snow off the driveway. The forecast for the next week or so is more or less snow every day, nothing spectacular, but consistent.

It is Friday night approaching midnight. Carol woke up a little combative but settled into a pretty good day after that. I look over at her birthday roses and see that they are wilting. In all honesty my care of them was perfunctory, adding a little new water every couple of days and ignoring whatever was in the little packets the florist had instructed me to add to the water.

That thought leads me to what follows.

Years ago, when we took a car trip to Salem and Concord, Massachusetts, the home turf of a number of my favorite writers, I bought a souvenir T-shirt. On its front, the face that Nathaniel Hawthorne said belonged to the ugliest man he had ever seen, stares out under one of his strongest recommendations. "Simplify," it says.

With that word, Henry David Thoreau preaches his antidote to what he perceived to be the misery of his society where he saw the masses leading lives of "quiet desperation," suffering from the disease William Wordsworth had earlier diagnosed in a sonnet as wasting our powers with too much "getting and spending."

All of which is an unnecessarily literary preface to the fact that I have simplified my life, not for the perhaps more substantial reasons of Thoreau and Wordsworth, but out of necessity. Given my caregiver responsibilities and time constraints, I cannot tend to many things I would otherwise take care of.

I do manage the getting and spending in the mundane

terms of the household cash ebb and flow, paying bills, and keeping an eye on disbursements from my IRA. I recognize that both Henry and William had more fundamental ideas in mind, but this is where I am now. I do the cooking, laundry, and necessary cleaning. Otherwise, I subcontract or ignore the rest.

So as winter approached, instead of hauling out the leaf blower, I contracted with the local company that I used to hire only to finish the massive job of clearing away the mountain of leaves layering our heavily treed property.

I gave up keeping the bird feeders stocked. Our feathered friends were on their own.

For now, I will probably continue to snow blow the driveway, but if that turns out to be too time-consuming or onerous, I will hire help for that chore.

These extra expenses are not particularly troublesome since our entertainment budget, once fairly healthy, has now dropped to about zero. Instead of going out to eat or attending concerts and movies, money goes to do things I no longer feel I can do.

As with so many other changes, this one parallels how I have come to see myself. I am primarily a caregiver. Responsibilities associated with that role take priority over everything else.

I get no gratitude from Carol, nor should I expect any. I suppose the dog is happy that she is fed and let out to do her business as necessary. Friends tell me they respect what I am doing, but they cannot have any idea of what that really means.

I'm not talking about needing a pat on the back. After all, keeping Carol at home with me for as long as I can has been, and remains, my deeply held preference.

I am only holding up a figurative mirror to look at myself, to see what I have become through the lens of what I can and cannot do.

What comes back to me from that activity is clear enough.

What follows, though, remains to be seen.

Super Bowl Sunday night after a snowy weekend requiring several sessions behind the snowblower to clear the driveway. I watched the game on the big screen TV downstairs while Carol slept. Because of my interest in football, she sometimes tried to watch games with me, but she never really succeeded in sharing my enjoyment. I don't think she objected to the violence of the game, for she loved watching boxing. I suppose learning the rules and strategies required more effort than she wanted to invest.

The question now, of course, is moot.

We are both accommodating ourselves to the hospital bed. As advertised, it makes certain activities, such as raising Carol to a sitting position, easier. The sleeping surface is considerably wider than that which the sofa offered, and Carol sometimes gets herself into oddly angled positions, but for the most part she does sleep well enough in it.

I have now, however, discovered one of the reasons I delayed for so long in obtaining the bed, and why in spite of its advantages, I am still unhappy with it.

I thought my reluctance was based on the presence of the bed introducing an unwanted change in the feel of our shared living space.

That much was, and is, true.

But I now understand that there is a deeper level.

When we were both sleeping on the sofa, it was possible for me to position myself in such a way as to be able to be in close physical proximity. Our sofa is an L-shaped sectional. Carol occupied and slept on one leg of it. During the day, aside from attending to her needs, I did not spend much time on the sofa. But sometimes, I would bend myself around the corner of the sectional so that I could put my arm around her.

I cannot do that with her in the bed. It is placed against the wall opposite the sofa. I can sit on the arm of the sofa and reach over or through its railing but doing so is awkward.

Before, I typically slept on my leg of the sofa with my head away from her and my feet encroaching into the corner section. In the mornings, I would awaken, reverse my position so that my upper body was now on that corner section, and I could reach her to hold her hand, or stroke her cheek or hair. Sometimes she objected to this attention, but most times she accepted it happily, or so it seemed.

I now see that my ability to do that preserved the fiction that we were still living as we had, in the shared intimacy of husband and wife.

The bed has removed that fiction.

In it, she the patient, I the caregiver.

Woke up to a steady but light snow this morning. I decided to forego my usual Sunday morning jaunt to the store to pick up the New York Times *along with a muffin for Carol and whatever else we might need until I do a full grocery shopping trip. Just didn't want to deal with the snow although there wasn't that much accumulation. Read the paper online and gave Carol her ordinary breakfast.*

It's Sunday night as I write this. Watched Victoria *and* Queen Elizabeth's Secret Agents. *Carol, of course, dozed in her bed. Even the dog chose her bed instead of coming into the TV room with me. I'm getting used to these solo television watching occasions.*

But not happily.

Every once in a while, a line from some source will jump into my consciousness for no particular reason, or at least no reason I can identify.

That happened yesterday. I don't now recall what I was doing at the moment, but whatever it was I am fairly certain it had nothing to do with this sentence that flashed itself into my consciousness.

"So we beat on, boats against the current, borne back ceaselessly into the past."

That is the last line of F. Scott Fitzgerald's *The Great Gatsby*.

Although decades ago, I taught that book in an American Literature survey course, and although I admire it immensely, I have not thought about it in a very, very long time.

And yet, yesterday, that line popped into my consciousness. No, that's not exactly right. I did not have all the words, or even most of them. Rather, I recalled that the novel ended with something about a boat and rowing. I then did what we all do nowadays, rather than digging the book off whatever shelf it is now on, I Googled something like "Gatsby rowing."

And the line appeared.

This is not the place, nor do I have the energy, to suggest the line's relationship to the novel, why Nick Carraway, the narrator, is made to say it. Rather, taken out of its context it speaks powerfully to me in my situation.

It captures the pull backward that I deal with numerous times every day whenever something in our house reminds me with considerable force of the life we have left behind, be it the Victorian pictures of a girl reading a book on the wall in the downstairs bathroom, or the wooden sign announcing "Baths 5 Cents" on the wall of the upstairs bathroom, both chosen and installed by Carol, the one expressing her own particular version of feminism informed by her love for reading, the other a humorous reminder of her historical sensibility.

And of course, there is the more serious pull of those moments, far enough between, but powerful when they occur, when with some gesture, or word or two, Carol for a moment is again herself.

That happened a night or two before, and again last night, when on each occasion, she said in a very quiet voice, "I love you." I permitted myself, each time, to savor the moment. It would have been wiser, perhaps, to discount it, to understand its ephemeral nature, how impossible it is to be sure of its significance. She might even have been declaring her love for the me in her memory rather than the me in front of her.

But of course, emotions trump rational thought.

And so, for the moment, I let myself in my little rowboat be borne back by the current into our shared past.

The larger question is how hard do I want to row against that current. Do I, in fact, want to beat it and begin to leave that past behind me?

Fitzgerald is no doubt suggesting that so to do is impossible. We may beat against the current, but it will prevail. Perhaps we will make a little progress, only to be thrown back.

Thus far, I see Fitzgerald's words as an accurate representation of my situation. The metaphor is apt: rowing against the current is an arduous business, forward movement bought with the expenditure of considerable muscular energy. That thought reminds me of the time my father took me fishing in a rented rowboat on Sheepshead Bay off the south coast of Brooklyn, and only with great difficulty rowed us back against the outgoing tide. Shortly thereafter, he bought an outboard motor he would attach to the rented boats.

For me, now, it would be the expenditure of emotional rather than muscular energy to provide the movement away from the past.

I can also see that if the past is dominated by pain or disillusionment, as may be the case for Nick when he offers these words, then the point is the difficulty of putting some distance between you and the occasion of that pain or disillusionment.

Moving from a painful past is complicated when the pain is, as is often the case, tied up with something very good.

Which is where I am.

I do not want to forget my past with Carol.

But remembering it, and knowing how it is irretrievably gone, is its own kind of pain.

Nor do I know what exactly I am rowing toward.

To Hoist or Not to Hoist and Carol's Journals

Another deceptively warm day, snow melting, sun out. You'd almost think spring was around the corner. But it is mid-February in northern Michigan, and snow is predicted for early next week.

Today was, in fact, Valentine's Day. A few cards for us, or Carol alone, came in the mail the past few days. Carol and I never paid much attention to this contrived holiday, and so it did not generate any feelings in me. I suppose I could say that for us every day was Valentine's Day.

I have started to listen to classical music streaming from WSHU, a station from Connecticut I used to tune to when we lived on Long Island. It is playing in my ears now as I write. I don't recognize the piece, but it has a strong romantic feel, perhaps in honor of the day.

Music just ended. It was from Wagner's "Tristan und Isolde."

The ebb and flow of this disease continues, oscillating within very narrow parameters.

The therapists, physical and occupational, were back today, and again made some limited progress. They got Carol on her feet and into the transport chair, then wheeled her into the kitchen with the idea of having her stand holding onto the sink. When that seemed a step too far, they settled for having her eat her lunch, a protein bar, while sitting in the chair, and then back to her bed.

During these proceedings, I assisted both verbally and physically. When she was sliding out of the chair, I helped hoist her back up.

Tired. Enough for tonight. Resume tomorrow.

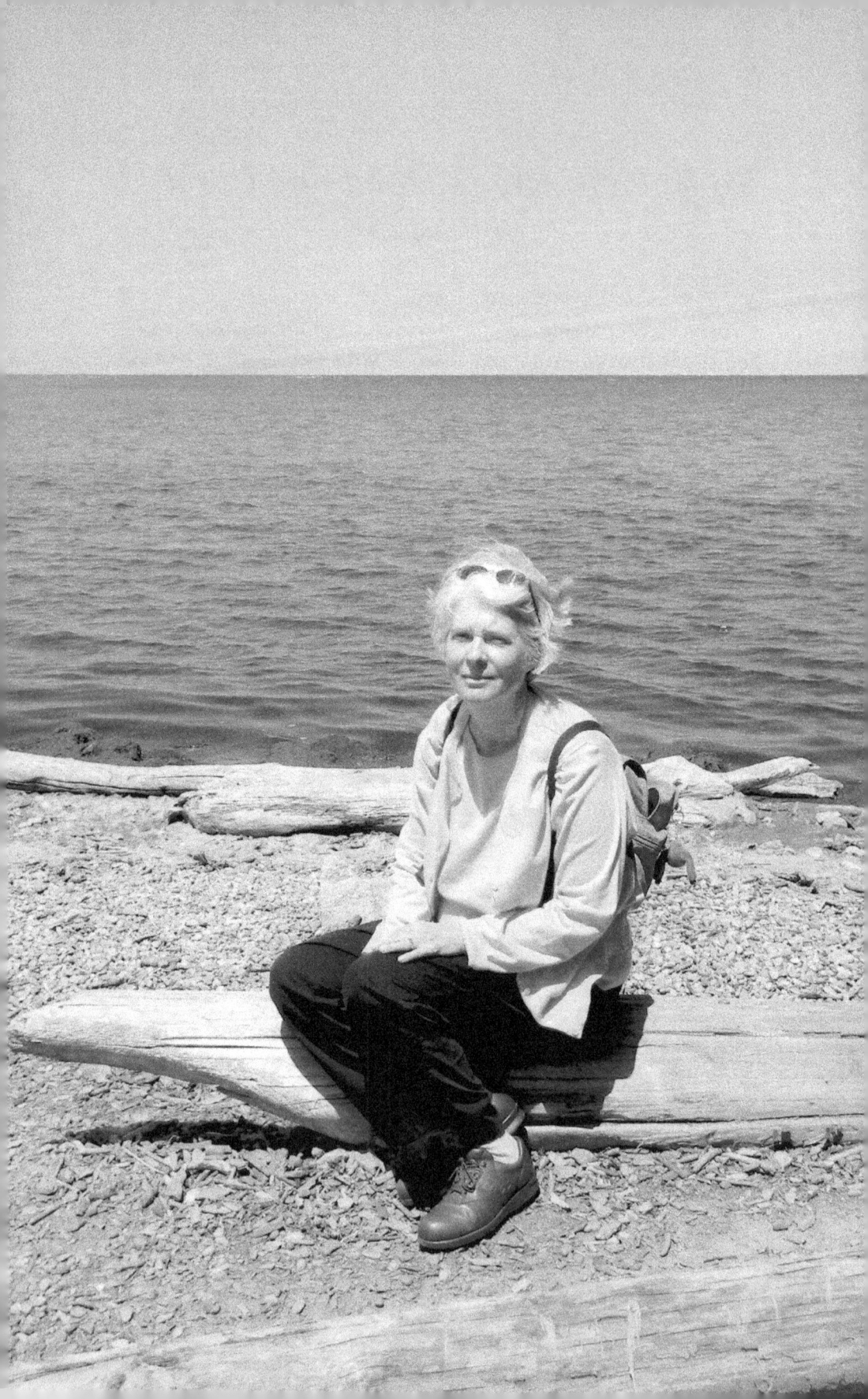

In the library this afternoon after snow shower this morning.

Teacher has brought kindergarten kids into the library and is offering a lesson on Washington whose birthday will be celebrated in a few days. She ends by saying that she shares the same birthday, and wouldn't it be nice if she were elected the first woman president.

I am thinking about chairs in the context of the narrow parameters in which Carol's disease seems to move.

This morning after giving Carol her breakfast in her bed, I served myself mine sitting at the kitchen table. I looked up, across the table, at her empty chair. That image prompted me to remember my watching television last night alone in the green room, sitting in one of the matching upholstered recliners.

Those chairs contrast in my mind with the transport chair, an imposition into our household necessary to deal with the effects of Carol's disease. With heroic efforts, it might be possible to touch the top of the narrow band within which she is living so that I will be able on a regular basis to get her in and out of that chair.

The therapists are moving in that direction. They are not sure that they will be able to get to the point where I alone can do what now requires both of them, namely, to move her from her bed into that chair.

They suggest a device called a Hoyer hoist, which would literally lift her out of bed and deposit her into the chair. Once in the chair, perhaps supplemented by another recommended device called a pommel cushion, which would prevent her from slouching down and off, I would be able to wheel her to the breakfast table.

And the TV room where we could watch television together. Sort of.

<<< In Old Mission, ca. 2002.

For she would not, I am sure, really process the visual images on the TV screen, although she might do better with the audio.

That might be enough for her to get some enjoyment out of the upcoming Kentucky Derby, advertisements for which have already started airing. Carol, an excellent rider herself, loved horses and horse races. We used to take walks along a dirt road next to a fenced-in pasture, and she always had an apple or two with her to offer to the horses, who would trot over to us and take the fruit out of her hand. All of that was pretty extraordinary for this city boy to witness, whose experience with horses was of the wooden variety at the merry-go-round in Coney Island.

Sunday night. I alternated my TV viewing between my continuing binge watching of Peaky Blinders, *a kind of British* Sopranos, *and the usual* Victoria, *which just manages to be on the right side of the balance between historical drama and soap opera.*

Some time ago I came across Carol's handwritten journals in which she recorded her progress on the fiction she was writing. For reasons I now will never be able to ask her about, there is a huge gap in these documents. Both start about 2005 and continue into the next year. One stops there while the other picks up for a few pages seven years later in 2012.

That there are two journals essentially covering the same period does not surprise me. I long ago understood how Carol's difficulty with organization and fear of losing things produced duplication of storage. Even when she worked with word processing, I could not convince her to simply save the new version under the same file name with which she had opened the document. Instead, she would save each version with a slightly different name by adding a number or date, thus making each a new file. The result was a long list of files that were essentially the same except for a little new material in each.

So, the two journals pretty much covering the same ground is, if anything, predictable. I did find them in different locations. But the gap in the one before picking up again seven years later is not explained by this organizational difficulty.

To the best of my recollection those intervening seven years were unremarkable, nothing of any import having occurred during that time. So why she abandoned and then returned to that journal will have to remain a mystery. Also unanswered is why the continuation did not last very long.

What I found most interesting besides this gap were the comments concerning her aspirations as a writer.

I had known, of course, that Carol wanted to succeed as a writer. I did not know the intensity of her ambition, revealed in her journals. I probably took too literally her sometimes expressed concerns as to how she would handle celebrity as a writer should it come her way.

Which, I now more clearly understand, did not mean she didn't want the recognition. She did.

But she also wanted to use her writing to document the wrongs she saw. I was struck by a passage in the journal where she argued with her mother's insistence on always being "nice." The world was not nice, Carol thought, and her stories would be honest in representing that fact.

In lesser hands, this motivation could well lead to failure as a writer by letting the message sink the story. But Carol was too good a storyteller to let that happen. Her stories do deal with the harsh realities of disadvantaged people, whether they be unsuccessful farming families, migrant Mexican workers, or, and most especially, Native Americans. But they do not preach. They just reveal.

I was also unaware of how she struggled to do what she loved, which was to write. In the journals, which for the most part say nothing about me, she expresses her frustration that I would never understand her difficulty overcoming her attention-deficit disorder. I simply do not remember much discussion of that problem, perhaps a few passing remarks, widely scattered.

But apparently she wrestled mightily with it. The journals provide some support for that idea in the sense that the notes meant to pull together her ideas for her fiction were more like stabs rather than a smoothly developed progression.

I guess I did not pick up on whatever clues I might have because the product she produced was so damned good that I just assumed it did not require more than any good writer's self-editing skills.

It might also explain, although there are certainly other explanations, why she could never master longer canvases, such as a novel, or the nonfiction book she so much wanted to write about Sarah Lane, who upon the death of her husband became the first woman keeper of the local lighthouse. Carol did a tremendous amount of research but could not get a handle on the possible shape of the book. She sought my help, and I tried to organize her material for her. But probably because it was my approach rather than her own, that did not work.

I suggested she try to write it into a novel, thinking the fictional approach might be easier. I don't believe she ever started down that road.

Of course, I now see what I didn't see, and which, for her own reasons, she did not make clear to me.

There is also just a hint of the predictable friction that can occur between two writers who happen to also be lovers. I don't think we competed. Our egos were too strong to feel challenged by the other. Rather, because we were so in love with each other, critiquing each other's work could be problematic. Not that we wouldn't offer honest assessments. We did.

But we didn't always agree with those assessments.

And finally, though, we each sought the approval of the

other. If nobody else in the world liked what we wrote, it would be nearly enough if the other of us did.

I had to add that qualifier *nearly*.

But the point remains.

Among all the qualities of our relationship I miss, our shared passion for writing is one that leaves a huge void.

After another faux spring day with temperatures approaching sixty degrees, winter decided to return today with a mixture of freezing rain and snow predicted for tomorrow as we head into the weekend.

A quiet evening. Carol has been sleeping a lot today, as has the dog. I couldn't get interested in anything on television, nor did I feel like reading.

So, since it is too early for me to go sleep, I might as well write for a while.

I am feeling unusually lonely. Nothing dramatic has changed to account for this mood.

But if not dramatic, there seem to be a few contributing factors. One is a discussion I had with the physical and occupational therapists yesterday.

They pushed me hard toward ordering that hoist, the device that would enable me to lift Carol off the bed and into a wheelchair. They had succeeded once again in getting Carol on her feet for a bit and then into the chair. But when they tried to get her to sit more upright, the situation deteriorated. Carol slouched and I had to help pull her up and off the chair, so they could maneuver her back into the bed.

Perhaps that is why they started to promote the idea of the hoist. They described how good it would be for Carol to again move around the house, albeit in the chair.

That had some appeal for me.

But accommodating this device in our living space would require creating space for it. It will not fit in the room where the bed now is without removing some furniture. The likely candidate would be to detach one leg of our L-shaped sectional.

Then where would that go?

I found myself losing myself in these very mundane considerations.

And as usual, they were masking my deeper concerns. Still, I agreed to have them begin the ordering process.

After they left, the mother/daughter housecleaning team came and after they were pretty much done, I talked with them about the hoist. They've been coming to us for a long time, and I was quite comfortable discussing this matter with them, as they were easy about offering their views.

We considered several possible landing places for the sectional piece. But for each there was a problem, a narrow doorway here, too many turns on the staircase there, another narrow doorway upstairs leading to the unused room that had been Carol's office.

No doubt professional movers could work something out.

But these issues, I realized, were not primarily what was bothering me. Upon calmer reflection, I did not see the huge advantage that the therapists had envisioned. Even if I were able to use the device to get Carol into the chair, she would no doubt initially, and perhaps permanently, resist the process. With her intense fear of falling, being suspended in the hoist, persistent fear, if not outright panic, is quite likely.

In short, I did not see enough positive outcomes to make this lift idea attractive. I also realize that the therapists, through their own comments, see obtaining this device as a way of justifying continued Medicare support because they would be training me to use it.

Without that justification, and with no clear sign that their efforts were producing a quantifiable result, they might not be able to continue getting paid.

That is a problem. But not a reason to agree to getting a device for which I really see issues on the one hand, and not much to be gained, on the other.

I relayed my decision not to get the hoist to the therapists.

They came one more time to have me sign off on their ending their efforts.

I did so with some relief. The therapists' push for progress, justified perhaps in their minds as necessary for them to provide service, had influenced my judgment as to what was right and good.

For Carol.

For me.

At this time.

Loomings

Late Sunday morning. Carol is drowsing, almost asleep, then sort of awake. I've been to the store to pick up the Times *and Carol's Sunday breakfast treat of a blueberry muffin. After breakfast, she was convinced her mother was waiting for her to go to church. Telling her that her mother is in assisted living and not expecting her did not pull her into the here and now. She was fixed in some past moment. Her eyes are now closed, and then she calls my name. Sometimes she does that just, it seems, to assure herself that I, or maybe her memory of me, is around. I expect she will fall fully asleep.*

I've got classical music playing from the local public radio station in part to counter the wind outside and in part to provide background while I write for a while.

This morning I did what I always do upon rising from my bed on the couch. I moved the pillow and blanket out of sight.

Carol, eyes closed, is yelling at some voice or action in her head. Nothing I can usefully respond to.

Until today, I did not pause to think why I do this. On a day when I expect a visit from somebody, moving my sleeping material out of sight makes a little bit of sense although I am sure my visitor would not care one way or another.
But I would.
And that is the point, I realized today, and explains why even on a Sunday when nobody is expected, I repeat this minor straightening up activity.
I want the room to look as much as possible as it always did. That is not a new thought, of course. But until today, I had not applied it to my morning routine. Just another of the ways, big and small, I continue to struggle with my refusal

to abandon the Carol that was. Perhaps readers will tire of hearing that refrain, but it is the context within which I live, and it will poke its head out, unbidden and unwanted.

A piece of music has just ended, the wind continues to make noise outside, and Carol's eyes are closed. The dog is sprawled asleep on the floor.

I realize that writing now as we move into Sunday afternoon is a good countermeasure to my loneliness.

I can at least commune with myself.

This struggle between the then and now took a very particular shape these past few weeks. Looming ahead was my grandson's bar mitzvah on Long Island, New York.

The word "looming" might sound inappropriate.

But it is not.

It focuses quite precisely on this then/now dichotomy.

I pause. The English professor in me objects. "Dichotomy" is not the right word. It suggests a division, a clean separation between two opposites. Night and day. Good and evil.

My then/now situation is not so clear. It is this lack of clarity that argues for the applicability of "looming," which suggests an event or circumstance you would rather avoid. I will try to explain how the word fit this upcoming event, which presented me with a decision I would rather not have had to make, but one I could not avoid. Whatever I did would leave me unhappy.

I could not simply book a flight as I did two years ago when I attended the bar mitzvah of the older brother of the one whose rite was coming up. Then, I was able to leave Carol at her mother's house while I flew to New York. Her mother was being taken care of round the clock by several caregivers, and Carol was still functional enough to not strain that setup.

Her mother is now in a care facility, so that option was not available. This time I would need to find a respite facility for Carol where I would leave her alone, and I would return to an empty house.

Of course, she would not be literally alone, and the house would only be empty until she returned the next day.

This scenario in my mind was a precursor, perhaps, of what awaits me and her down the road.

Still, I shoved these negative thoughts, whom I imagine to be a shrouded figure in a black robe, sort of like death itself without the scythe, into a closet. I shut the door and began working to make this trip possible.

I soon discovered that respite facilities do not take reservations because their business models, reasonably enough, seek to have all beds occupied all the time.

But with some difficulty, I found a facility that could be persuaded by a nonrefundable deposit to hold a bed open. Because I was unable to book a flight much in advance, I decided to drive. My route would take me through Canada into upstate New York with a stop in Syracuse overnight with very good friends, and then on to Long Island. I would stay for two or three days with other friends whom I've known since college, and on the grounds of whose house Carol and I were married thirty-two years ago.

I booked the dog into the kennel we use, arranged to have a hospital bed installed in the facility for Carol, reminded myself that I would have to put a hold on our mail and stop the newspaper delivery. I made sure I had my abbreviated passport for the passage into Canada, and even dug out a handful of Canadian currency from the last time we had taken this route.

The prospect of a long car trip, something I always enjoy, the stops with friends, and, of course, the celebration itself kept the door of that closet shut.

The black-robed figure scratched and scratched.

Then one last problem arose and forced that door open.

I got a call from the nurse at the hospital who was arranging for the ambulance to take Carol to the facility. It would cost, she said, eleven hundred dollars each way, an outrageous amount for a twenty-four-mile trip.

Ignoring that shrouded figure, now fully out of the closet, I got in touch with the new chief of our local fire department, which has an ambulance, to see if he could provide transportation. I had made his acquaintance some time ago when I enlisted his help to move Carol from the couch onto the hospital bed that had just been set up in our living room. He had said, then, to call when I needed help. I knew not to take that statement too literally, and that asking for the use of the department's ambulance for a nonemergency trip would leave it unable to respond to an actual emergency.

It was a long shot.

Of course, with many apologies the chief said he couldn't leave his department in such an untenable position.

Further efforts to find an alternative, private or public, came up empty.

I could have sucked it up and agreed to pay the outrageous price.

But I could not convince myself to do that. The shrouded figure had a bony finger on my shoulder.

He had won.

And I decided to stay home.

I am afraid that some family members have concluded that I did not make the trip because I could not afford it.

That is not right, but I understand why they might think so since I did tell them that the exorbitant transport fee was what decided me against going.

If the situation were as simple as paying the fee would have caused me and Carol to live on peanut butter sandwiches for a month, then the fee would have been the cause.

But that was not the case.

If, like two years ago, I could have comfortably left Carol with her mother, both of them being taken care of by her family, I most likely would have unhappily paid the fee.

But that was not the case.

I could not comfortably leave Carol, not even remotely so.

The fee tipped the balance.

Here's why.

One morning while I was wrestling with this situation, I walked back into the living room after attending to some minor household chore, and saw that Carol was visibly upset, trembling and near tears. As I approached her, she reached out, and said, "Oh, you're back."

I leaned over her bed, and she took my arm and pulled it to her. We sat that way for some time.

And then I was able to get up and prepare our breakfasts.

It is probably hard for those not in my situation to fully grasp both the poignancy of that little scene and its ambiguity. In terms of the latter, I accepted that she recognized me for her present Steve rather than her memory of me. Maybe that is false. But I don't think so. And in any case, that is how I perceived it.

That made leaving her in a respite facility, as a precursor of a permanent move to such a place, like getting a kick in the stomach.

Or consider the following conversation from a few days later.

I came back into the living room from the kitchen singing nonsense words off key.

I do this whenever my mood dictates. It's my way of being cheery.

Carol looked up and with some effort formed the word "singing."

"Yes," I answered. "But I don't sing on key." I paused. "You like to sing, don't you?"

She smiled, and we were, for the moment, together in the here and now. I pushed the envelope to see how far we could go.

"When we first moved here," I continued, "you joined a chorus in town."

She looked puzzled.

"Did I?" she murmured.

"Yes," I replied.

And then we were lost somewhere between now and then, her memory having failed to bring up what was, in truth, a minor episode, as for reasons I no longer recall she did not stay with that singing group very long.

I turned the conversation back to a firm foothold in the now.

"I've got a scone for breakfast for you."

"Scones, they're good."

"And I went to the co-op and got you the pear juice you like."

That brings a big smile, and for the moment, we are back together in the same time frame, hanging on to a shared memory.

And so it goes, from moment to moment, and day to day, like spent waves approaching our footprints in the damp sand and then with the next incursion of the incoming tide washing them away.

Going to New York would have yanked me back to dry sand beneath my feet.

Perhaps a good thing.

But I wasn't ready for it.

On A Date Certain

Tuesday night. A long, tiring day that began with clearing six inches of snow off the driveway and then driving to town for weekly grocery shopping. I've decided to add back the co-op grocery store, which in the interest of economy of motion, I had been skipping. I stop there now for the organic veggies, interesting juices, such as blueberry, and, of course, the freshly baked cookies.

My decision to return to the co-op for part of our grocery needs was motivated only in part by what can be purchased there in contrast to the regular grocery store. The fact is I had never been as enthusiastic about shopping there as Carol was. She placed far more emphasis on being careful about the food she ingested than did I. And prices at the co-op are high.

I recognize that my initial motivation to shop at the co-op again was to say hello to our nephew who now works there. He had just graduated from Michigan State, and I wanted to say to him something like, "See what a first-class college education gets you, unpacking and shelving food stuffs." I know, of course, he is just trying to earn the money he will need to live on when he begins his unpaid internship working for a local politician.

So, my intention was to stop there once, deliver that line, have a laugh, and that would be it. As it turns out, his schedule and mine did not mesh, and I did not see him there after all.

But something strange happened when I re-entered the store after not having been in it for perhaps a year.

I felt a positive vibe.

So, the next week, and the one after, I continued stopping there, just for a few items, while continuing to do the bulk of my shopping as before. My attitude toward the store had changed. It felt right to be there.

And then I understood. Shopping there increased my hold on the then, on Carol as she had been, pushing back for the while against the inevitable imposition of the now.

This made more sense when I told Carol the cookie she was having for dessert or the juice she was drinking came from the co-op. She quite clearly responded with a big smile and a nod. Of course, she was saying without words, "I always told you how much I like to shop there."

Wednesday night. No appointments, no errands, no phone calls today. Carol in a reasonably good mood for most of the day. In the quiet I was able to attend to the business of being a writer, researching possible markets for my work, and that was a pleasant change.

Forecast is for snow tonight ending about noon when lunch with the guys minus one is scheduled. The one is now on the Alabama shore far removed from any threat of snow.

As I write this, I know the east coast is again being hammered. I hope my daughters and their husbands all got home safely.

Had I kept my plans to attend my grandson's bar mitzvah, I would probably be driving through this weather. Maybe there's some god looking down and declaring let's give him a break. He could use one.

I do worry about my own well-being. Well, of course, I do. But for me if I wake up feeling a little off my feed, as they say around here, as I have done the past couple of days, I tell myself I just can't get sick. If I do, who is going to take care of Carol?

When I make my way carefully over the ice and snow to cross the road to get the newspaper or the mail I feel my hip to make sure I have my phone in case I take a header as I did last winter when my feet flew out from underneath me and I landed on my back. If I have my phone, I can call for help.

For Carol, that is.

I think of the picture posted on Facebook recently of a family member, a young man in his teens, smiling back at the camera, his arm in a cast from a fall on the ice.

I simply can't afford to be sick or injured.

Of course, something would be worked out. But I worry, nonetheless.

Carol as she usually does is sleeping on her back, snoring loudly. The dog has risen from her bed and wandered into the kitchen. Sometimes she chooses to sleep by her food dish. Maybe she thinks doing so will somehow cause the bowl to be filled. If I am writing about the dog that means the well has dried up tonight and I will just stop for now.

Back at it on a Thursday evening. Day began, again, with clearing the driveway in time for arrival of caregiver relief and to enable me to keep my weekly lunch date during which we had a good conversation about guns and the Second Amendment. Somehow from deep in my memory I recalled that in Boston in 1637 that city's government disarmed a group of dissenters from the prevailing religious establishment. I retained that factual nugget from my research years ago for a historical novel I wrote but never sold.

Nurse practitioner came later in the afternoon and found that Carol continues in fine physical shape.

Before the nurse practitioner examined Carol, we had a conversation concerning the meeting scheduled for tomorrow in my house to discuss care strategies. The participants will be the supervisors of the hospital's private duty program, the two aides who provide respite relief for me under that program, and a nurse who occasionally makes home visits, as she did last Friday to cut Carol's nails.

In anticipation of the meeting, since it is deliberately being scheduled in my house so as to enable me to participate and provide my perspective, I wrote out what I would like these professionals to know.

To wit. It is my firm intention to keep Carol living with me in this house for as long as I can. From that intention everything else flows. First, I need respite relief from my 24/7 caregiver responsibilities. Thus, the primary help I seek from the aides is providing me time to do what I need or want to do. In addition, I appreciate the aides assuming certain tasks that I cannot do well, such as giving Carol a bath and washing her hair. One of the aides does that job much better than I can now manage, and I have no ambition to add that chore to my caregiver skill set. Finally, I am happy to have trained medical people here regularly who can alert me to problems I might otherwise not notice or be aware of.

When I leave Carol in the hands of the aides, I expect upon my return I will find her safe and her needs well attended to. All else is extra. If Carol is sleeping, as she often is, and the aide wants to do some minor housecleaning, good, go for it. I certainly won't object. If the aide wants to try to interact with Carol, read to her, play music, or just chat, good. But if Carol is not interested, that is fine as well.

In the library after the meeting. Young kids, perhaps first graders, are being coached into producing a puppet show version of "Jack and the Beanstalk." I find it somehow refreshing to be in the presence of such youthful exuberance, the giggles of delight. Would that the world were so innocently delightful.

But it, especially my world, is not.

The meeting went well. We covered the points I had laid out, moved on to an extensive conversation concerning products I should buy to provide better hygienic care, and discussed strategies for improving interpersonal interaction with Carol, based on the aides' experiences and what perspectives I could provide.

"Fee fi fo fum, I smell the blood of an Englishman" comes across the room in the teacher's voice reaching for, but not

139

quite arriving at, a basso tone as the show draws to its close, followed by humdrum chore of taking attendance.

We also went over Carol's meds with the idea of perhaps eliminating some that may not any longer be useful or perhaps are now even counterproductive.

The kids are energized by the show, their high-pitched voices filling the sedate, book-lined aisles of the library. A happy convergence of young minds and the world-weary knowledge stored between the stiff bound covers of the books.

This morning I stopped by my office and saw, as I have countless times before, the old mechanical perpetual calendar on my desk. This is a device that provides three different wheels, one to change the day, one the date, and one the month. I have had it on my desk for probably close to half a century, stretching way back to precomputer days into the present, wherein I continued to turn those wheels to reflect the actual day.

Until I stopped doing so.

On Saturday, August 12, 2017, the day of my grandson's birthday, two days after our anniversary, and three days before my birthday, documenting the point I knew Carol would no longer be climbing the stairs to our bedroom. Actually, to be perfectly accurate, she had stopped dealing with the stairs some time before. Although I joined her in sleeping on the couch in our living room, I continued, as I do now, to climb those stairs every day for my morning shower and change of clothes as well as my occasional sit down at my desktop computer.

On one of those mornings, I stopped by my desk, looked at the perpetual calendar, and decided to leave it as it was that day August 12, 2017, the date certain when I acknowledged Carol's now insuperable aversion to those steps.

Another in a long line of concessions to the new now pulling away from the remnants of the old then.

The library is suddenly quiet as the kids have exited. The only sound now besides my fingers hitting the keys of my laptop is the hum coming from the ventilation system.

That fixed date contrasts conveniently with the meeting this morning, the focus of which was to make the new now as comfortable as possible. There was no talk of the future, probably because I had declared in my outline of what I thought we should talk about that my intention was to have Carol in the house with me as long as possible. Therefore, any talk of the future and the changes it might bring, for now, is premature.

As though that future is not to be.

A useful, but necessary, fiction.

Two Worlds and Not the Plot
of a Bad Novel

Saturday night and while Carol sleeps, I have been watching preseason baseball, my Dodgers playing the Cubs. Ordinarily, I would not write tonight, instead taking my usual one-day break to recharge the batteries. But tonight, changing metaphors, I sense that the well from which I draw my ideas is brimming with thoughts, feelings, and observations that need to be sorted out and expressed. I will try to get started, drop the bucket down, then pull it up, and see what's in it.

No doubt I will have to drop it in deeper, but this will do for now, just a few sentences for tonight.

Today has been emotionally exhausting. For several hours, I was literally in two different worlds.

This morning at precisely ten thirty, I clicked on a link that opened up a service that was about to stream my grandson's bar mitzvah on Long Island, New York. I had intended to be there, but for the combination of reasons I have already discussed, I canceled my plans to drive across country.

Instead of sitting in the temple among family, I was in my usual chair in the living room. I had made sure that we got moving early enough to take care of all morning chores, and Carol had fallen back asleep. I had toyed with the idea of setting up the laptop so she, too, could watch, but that was a silly foray back into the then whereas in the now Carol would in all likelihood not remember this young man whom we had not seen very often, and even if in the unlikelihood that she did, she no longer can process visual content on a screen.

Having abandoned the idea of sharing the event with her, my hope then was that she would sleep through it. That might sound unkind, but it was a practical concern.

She did.

And so I sat in my chair staring at my laptop screen while occasionally glancing at Carol and past her through our sliding glass door to a view of the back of our five-acre property that offers a sliver of East Bay beyond the trees. On this gray day, the sliver was dark blue tending toward black, and the trees were still bare of their leaves.

That scene contrasted sharply with the bright colors and textures of the interior of the temple, and as the streaming began I could hear the low murmur of the congregation out of the view of the camera, and watch as the final setup preparations were completed on the bima, the raised platform at the front of the sanctuary.

Thus, my two worlds.

That's a good enough start.

Sunday night after the first day of spring forward. Sun up an hour later and sets an hour later. Hereabouts dusk now approaches eight o'clock. By the peak of the summer, it will be another hour later.

Went to the store as usual this morning but the Times *hadn't been delivered yet. Read it online but missed the feel of paper. Rest of the day was, as usual, quiet and I had a chance to catch up on email including one related to my writing business. We'll see if that one bears fruit.*

The starkly different visuals of the bar mitzvah on my laptop screen versus the rural Michigan landscape outside my glass door only begin to explain the separation I experienced yesterday. There was, of course, and probably more intensely, the matter of the people on that screen dressed out in their fine clothes on the one hand and my bedridden wife on the other, while not forgetting the ever-present dog on the floor.

To be honest, I was not all that interested in the service itself. There's a reason why after my own bar mitzvah, I only attended services for necessary ritualistic occasions, primarily bar and bat mitzvahs. My attention to Judaism leans more heavily toward the cultural rather than the spiritual.

So, I waited for what I was most interested in seeing: the people who would be called up to participate at various times during the service. And most importantly, the bar mitzvah boy himself. As the rabbi and cantor opened the proceeding, the fixed camera providing the streaming captured the heads of my daughter and son-in-law. Then at different points, they and their older son would ascend the bima along with my other daughter, husband, and children. And the grandparents, not forgetting, of course, my ex-wife.

While I sat in my chair in Michigan.

It is hard to voice my feelings, to find the right words. I can say what I wasn't. I wasn't angry or sad. Nor was I happy. Perhaps a little curious, just to see them, how they presented themselves, especially the children.

I suppose bittersweet comes close to capturing my feelings. But only close.

I also felt, for what it is worth acknowledging, a confirmation of the decision I made, perhaps without full awareness of the implications, of my move a thousand miles away to northern Michigan.

Oh, I had good reasons then for the move. My New York money buying less expensive Michigan real estate. My lifelong distaste for suburban living. Carol's strong desire to return to her home turf. And maybe underlying all of that, my sense that no particular place claimed my affection.

Except the Brooklyn of my childhood.

And that is gone as is my youth. I have visited the Brooklyn of now, and I am not at all sure I would be happy there.

So, I reasoned, if that is not too strong a word, that since no place called to me, any place other than suburbia would do just fine.

That judgment was largely correct.

But only largely.

It did not hold up all that well while I was sitting in my

chair in Michigan watching my family celebrate the coming of age of my grandson.

While Carol, who always encouraged me to remain involved with my family, lay unaware in her bed.

My grandson did a fine job.

The camera did not provide close-ups.

If it did, I would have seen a confirmation of what I already know.

The final irony.

As if I needed proof of that ironic fact, it was articulated by my English cousin who spoke to me on the phone in the midst of the party later that afternoon.

"Stephen," she said, "I see a lot of you in Brandon."

Tuesday night, Carol not quite yet asleep. She had a difficult day, getting a bath and hair wash she, as the aide related to me, really did not want. I never witness these proceedings because they occur on my shopping day.

After a brief respite, winter has returned but so far only in the form of cold without much snow. Spring arrives next week, but northern Michigan is often indifferent to what the calendar says.

Today at my daughter Kerri's suggestion I downloaded an app that the kids use to video conference. Only they are not conferencing, they are doing what teenagers do as the name of the app suggests.

It is called Houseparty.

Apparently, Brandon socializes with his friends using this app. By arrangement this evening, we signed on. I held my phone in front of me as if I were taking a selfie, and on the other end the phone was so placed as to capture the image of whoever was in front of it. I congratulated Brandon on his successful performance, and he gave me the thumbs up sign. The conversation moved from him to his parents and then to Peter, his older brother. Brian, his father, wanted to know what the streaming showed. I explained the fixed camera provided a clear shot of the bima, but there were no close-ups, and only a sliver of the first row of the congregants showed up, sufficient, however, for me to see half of the top of his head.

Peter wanted to show me a couple of pages of Old English he had downloaded. I didn't learn why he was interested in this particular material, but I am aware that he is something of a history buff. He had written a translation above the Anglo-Saxon words. He has been invited to sign up for Honors English, the reading list for which includes "Beowulf," no doubt in translation. I don't know if that is why he went online to snatch this piece of that ancient language.

Peter's academic progress was the focus of the latter part of the conversation, and when it concluded I was again struck by the strange feelings engendered by this visit into this other world, the one inhabited by my daughters and their families. But in particular, I recalled with a familiar pang how fond Carol had been of Peter. She saw something in him that perhaps others had not, maybe his strong imagination so much like her own, or that he was just somewhat different, as she had been as a child. She saw that he, like herself, was drawn to the natural world with an unusual intensity.

I told her about this digital meeting and about Peter's exploration of Old English. She offered a small smile.

It might have been because she remembered.

More likely, it was just a socialized response, a product of her having been taught manners by her Southern mother.

The dementia has not stripped that bit of good breeding from her.

I suppose that is a good thing, but it is also a reminder of how much else has been lost.

A cold Thursday afternoon on the Ides of March, working in the library against the sound of books thumping as they are shelved. As is usually the case on the afternoons I come here, there are no other patrons.

I left Carol sleeping as she had been for the past few hours.
The aide will give her lunch when she awakens.

It seems like Long Island is reaching out to me to remind
me of my connections to it. Of course, this past weekend was
filled with the afterglow of Brandon's bar mitzvah, followed
on Monday evening by the session on Houseparty.

Then, last night, the phone rang as it has been with increasing frequency lately, one telemarketer after another, but
this time was different. My caller ID told me that it was an
old friend and colleague who lived in Fort Salonga, across
the road from me, and with whom I sometimes carpooled
and at others played tennis. Our daughters were of compa-
rable ages but did not develop strong ties with each other.

He called, he said, because last Friday at his retirement
party he spoke with mutual friends, heard from them about
Carol, and perhaps prodded by that sad news decided to get
back in touch with me.

And I am quite glad he did.

We had a warm, hour-long conversation. We spent some
time talking about Carol, but then moved on to catching
up, what our kids were doing, and what each of us was into
artistically. I was not surprised that his restless creativity
has led him to try writing plays, as well as to continue his
old passion for filmmaking. In the latter regard, he promised to send me copies of his recent documentaries.

But what sticks in my mind today as I sit here in the
library are the memories our conversation evoked of the college at which I worked for thirty-five years. He mentioned
a number of colleagues who were at the retirement party
whom I remember fondly and certainly would have enjoyed
seeing again.

He also told the story, which I must confess I did not
remember, of how I, as the Chair of Humanities, was instru-
mental in his being hired at the college. It's a great story,
involving his wearing a suit he had found on the road while

riding his motorcycle. He was wearing it when he strolled into my building, asked about a job, and was directed to my office. I told him he must find a way to write it up. Or maybe make it part of a film.

However, where all this leads, as it must, is to Carol.

For some ten years after his hiring, at that same college I met Carol, at that time what we in the education game called a nontraditional student, one well past the usual starting age.

She remembers—I should say used to remember—our meeting. She was working as a tutor in the writing center, for which I was administratively responsible. I came into the room, and as was my wont, sat on the teacher desk, lit a cigarette—still marginally acceptable in those days—and introduced myself.

And that is how this woman from rural northern Michigan, whose travels had brought her to Long Island, met this kid from Brooklyn.

It's hard not to make what follows not sound like a line from a bad novel, something which both of us would be ashamed to write. But nonetheless it is true.

Our attraction to each other, for whatever reason, was mutual and strong.

Strong enough that in memory it remains with as much strength as ever.

Even now.

Family Roots

Saturday afternoon, St. Patrick's Day, an unusual time for me to sit down to write, but some ideas began to percolate as I took a late morning shower and I want to at least get started seeing what they have to offer.

I am in my office, having just taken care of printing a check rather than using bill pay. The dog, as has become her wont, only came halfway upstairs. I have been trying to figure out why she does not follow me all the way up. This is not a major issue but rather an engaging puzzle. Assuming a high level of doggie intelligence, perhaps she understands that the upstairs is now foreign territory since we live so much on the main floor. On a lower level of cognitive functioning, maybe the dog treats my being upstairs the same as if I had left the house altogether. Or maybe she is just confused. Or she enjoys the sun coming through the window onto the landing.

I think I'll go with the last possibility.

Carol is sleeping but might waken soon, so I will just start heading in the direction that is forming in my head, with the intention of picking it up later tonight or tomorrow.

Today, I have on my well-worn Guy Noir sweatshirt. That fact is what demanded attention, and I will return to it, for it will bring me back to Carol.

But before that, mentioning St. Patrick's Day reminds me how my father—when he was on the job or in a social situation where he wanted to establish his presence—would refer to himself as "the big Irishman."

That self-characterization was factually questionable on two levels.

First, although unquestionably muscular, even powerfully built, at five feet nine and an estimated 190 lbs., he was not an especially "big" man. I am three inches taller and carry perhaps ten more pounds.

But I don't think of myself as "big."

My father chose to describe himself that way because he was not being literal minded, as I sometimes am. Rather, he was accurately indicating the enormous strength in that ordinary sized body. I have no argument looking at his statement from that perspective.

The second point is more interesting. Why call himself Irish?

To be sure he was born in County Armagh. But his parents were recent immigrants from Lithuania, and by the time he was about five they had moved the family to Manchester, England, where I still have an extended family of first cousins and succeeding generations.

So his Irishness was really just a matter of accidental place of birth. Nothing more.

And yet he liked to refer to himself that way. I never spoke with him about this preference, but in my own mind I thought I had it figured out. He must have calculated, consciously or not, that it was more acceptable in America, his adopted country, to which he had emigrated when he was twenty, to be Irish.

More acceptable than what?

Than Jewish.

He did tell stories of the anti-Semitism he had encountered growing up in Manchester. Or maybe he just thought the Irish assimilated here more easily.

That speculation, no doubt, revealed his lack of awareness of how Irish immigrants had been so scorned when they arrived here that the Know Nothing party rose to national prominence in the middle of the nineteenth century riding the vehemence of its anti-Irish, anti-Catholic agenda.

Carol is stirring. I will continue this.

Later the same afternoon. Shutterfly just gave me an

unwanted shock by sending an email, which opened up with a smiling Carol beaming back at me.

A promotion. Trying to sell its services. The picture was from eight years ago on our trip to California. The unexpected image struck me hard.

To resume and complete this long introduction to where I want to go today, while my father was an immigrant, my mother was born in New York, the daughter of Ukrainian parents. The Brooklyn in which I was raised was populated by immigrants of various ethnic and cultural persuasions trying to become American. Those of my generation had pretty much crossed over into that identity.

Carol's family background could not be more different. Her distant antecedents stretch back to the eighteenth century while the more recent ones have been farming on this peninsula since the middle of the nineteenth century.

If America with the exception of Native Americans is comprised of immigrants, some of them have been here a very long time.

Before I met Carol, I had never heard of Garrison Keillor, or *A Prairie Home Companion*, his radio variety show that presented his thoroughly Midwestern, what shall I call it, yes, a New York, Yiddish-based word, his thoroughly, unapologetic Midwestern *shtick*.

I became a fan, and thus the Guy Noir sweatshirt featuring one of his characters I am wearing today, serving as an emblem of how to some extent I merged my New York formed identity with Carol's. In other ways I adopted some Midwestern traits, much to the surprise of at least one of my brothers-in-law. I have learned to use a chain saw and split wood for our stove. I have somewhat expanded my knowledge of birds from the familiar pigeons of New York to the occasional eagle flying in our skies or the hummingbird at our feeder.

And Carol had learned to love New York when she lived

there, the diversity, the energy, the cosmopolitan perspective. She taught herself to navigate the subway system and to deal with the much greater intensity of interpersonal interactions in the city although I suspect she was never completely comfortable with them, as I never fully adjusted to Midwestern reserve and conflict avoidance.

Our thirty-six years together now almost equally divide between our respective geographical and cultural roots.

We are both different for having experienced our differences.

But one of us is losing awareness of who we've become and seems to be retreating back into who she had been.

As I loaded the dishwasher after supper this Tuesday evening, I saw on the windowsill the spent yahrzeit that I had lit a day late. I have the date marking the anniversary of my mother's death on my calendar, but over the weekend I had lost track. More importantly, however, and perhaps part of the reason the day slipped by unnoticed, is that Carol used to join me in this little candle lighting ceremony, yet another of her efforts to help me remember from whence I came.

Spring is trying to advance against the stubborn remnants of winter evident in the patches of snow still on the deck and grassy areas in front and back of the house. The roads, for now, are clear, and I sailed into town for my weekly shopping.

With the approach of warmer weather, we will soon hear the heavy thumping of diesel driven tractors as the farmers begin to prepare their orchards for the upcoming season. Accustomed as I had been to city noises, these sounds don't really bother me.

And I expect Carol rather enjoys them, that in her current condition they can remind her of her farm family roots. This is so even though as a young woman she had made up her mind that, as she has said countless times, she wanted to get out into the larger world.

She did, traveling west to Minnesota and east to New York, from this small rural community to the unspeakably larger environment of the metropolitan area. As my retirement approached, it seems as though she had seen enough and she felt again the pull of the land and its agricultural rhythms, and she made it clear that she wanted to return home.

And so we did.

And I learned the new rhythm. Up until then, I had long been accustomed to the structure of the academic calendar, fall semester, spring semester, summer, and back to the fall. What I experienced here was similar in having a defined pattern, a beginning, middle, and end contained within the boundaries defined by nature, and the different harvesting time of the local crops, primarily cherries first in the spring and ending with apples in the fall.

I am curious to see to what extent Carol this year will tune into the farming activity. I'm guessing that the noises of the farm vehicles will stir memories from the time when she drove them, especially the cherry shaker. Will she recall, as she so often did, that she was the first woman cherry shaker driver on the Peninsula?

I hope she does.

If her hold on the present is shaky and her ability to think about the future pretty well gone, her long-term memory can still provide ballast to steady her as she rides on the troubling waters of confusion.

Coming on midnight after a spectacularly uneventful day, uneventful that is with the exception of one phone call. Another physical therapist called, this one strongly recommended by the practice supervising Carol's care. Apparently, he has had good success with dementia patients. He will call again to set up an appointment.

He represents, perhaps, our last best shot.

As our equally divided bookcases represent our different reading tastes, so, too, did our approaches to our arable land. Carol's strong visual sense motivated her to plant flowers. She had definite ideas as to what colors she wanted and where she wanted them to be. Her last impulse in this direction was a desire for yellow daffodils. The spot that I suggested, to which she agreed, is a stretch of lawn between our two flowering crab apples. Creating a planting bed was more than I wanted to undertake in my present circumstances, so I hired a local husband and wife landscaping business to do the job.

Carol had one good season to enjoy that mass of yellow (with a few white sprinkled in for variety). This year, unless the new therapist has unexpected success that enables her to get to a window, she will not see them.

Although I appreciate the color of flowers, and when I was a kid in Brooklyn I found little patches of soil in our landlord's yard where I was permitted to grow zinnias, as an adult I prefer to plant things I can eat. So I have a vegetable garden in which I attempt, with mixed success, to grow beans, potatoes, tomatoes, and different other veggies in different years, such as corn, cucumbers, zucchini, and so forth.

Although I planted the vegetable garden, Carol enjoyed weeding it. In fact, she liked nothing better than to sit in the dirt attending to plants, be they flowers or vegetables.

I look over to the hospital bed where my farm girl wife sleeps, largely unaware at least for now of the impending planting season.

If she can no longer go to the outside, perhaps I can figure a way to bring it inside to her.

Late Monday night after a difficult day that has left me with little energy. Will get this section started and look to continue in the next day or two.

Having left Carol dozing late morning, I went upstairs to my office computer to work on Quicken in anticipation of a meeting with our tax preparer the end of the week. I came down after about half an hour with a basket of laundry. Glanced at Carol as I passed by.

She looked a little restless, and I thought about seeing if she wanted lunch. Took the laundry downstairs, dumped it in the machine, and started the wash.

I remembered that I had intended to call the dentist to schedule my regular cleaning. Her office had sent an automated phone reminder yesterday on a Sunday. Unusual, but effective. I felt I should take care of that. We have a landline phone downstairs, but I decided to call from upstairs.

I came back from upstairs into the living room.

Carol was not lying as she had been.

Her whole body was shaking. I approached her on the bed to ask what was the matter.

That was when I saw the blood coming out of her mouth, mixed with spittle, accompanied by a gurgling sound.

Stupidly I asked her again what was the matter. Of course, she did not respond. More blood came out of her mouth. I found a washcloth, wet it, and wiped her mouth as the blood continued to spill out.

I talked to her. She did not respond. I took her hand, and she held on to it.

The shaking stopped. So did the blood.

But still she did not speak.

I sat with her, holding her hand. Her eyes kept moving from left to right, but I am not sure she was actually seeing anything.

When I was sure the shaking and the blood were not going to start up again, I called the practice and described the incident to the nurse, who said it sounded as though Carol had had another seizure. The blood, she said, likely came from Carol biting her tongue. She wanted to know if I wanted to have her taken to the hospital. I was not sure what the right thing to do was. I said I wanted somebody to check her out. What I meant was I did not know how to accomplish that, but that was what I wanted. The nurse said she would move people around and send somebody out.

Enough for tonight. I need sleep.

The Insistence of Hope

My old friend the deity I named George decided to pay me a visit today, either to distract me from the serious business of Carol's seizure or to just pile on, I'm not sure which. Either, no doubt, would amuse him.

When I saw the message from eBay in my inbox, I recognized George's hand, for that message informed me that my recent order had to be canceled because of a problem with the shipping address.

Yes, there was a problem, but not with the address.

I hadn't ordered the item. When I went to my eBay account, I saw the recent history of items I had checked out. But, of course, I didn't recognize them, for I had not trafficked on eBay in quite some time.

Most of my morning was thus spent, all the while keeping one eye on Carol, doing the protect the security of my account dance, the steps for which I am now familiar with from previous experiences with Amazon and my email account.

I finished all that just in time to give Carol lunch before the aide came, releasing me to go to town for my weekly shopping. So here I am at the end of a very long day, trying to pick up where I left off concerning the seizure.

The nurse practitioner came out within an hour or less from the onset of the seizure. She checked Carol's vitals and looked to see responses to visual and audio stimuli. She snapped her fingers near Carol's eyes or asked her to move her head toward the right. Carol's responsiveness was limited. She then, with my help, took a blood sample, which she would drop off at the hospital in town to see if a cause for the seizure would be revealed. Her best guess is that the seizure was just a product of the progress of the disease and probably not caused by stress as had been suggested when she had the first seizure in December.

Today, the lab test results reported nothing that would have caused the seizure, and Carol seems mostly recovered. Last night, she had trouble eating because of her injured tongue and would tolerate only cottage cheese. But today, she had her usual breakfast and half a sandwich for lunch. The aide reported that Carol resisted a full bath, permitted some washing, and went back to sleep. She roused for a full supper, including a large cookie for dessert, and then went back to sleep.

I'm assuming that tomorrow, she will be fully back to what I now know as her normal state.

Lost in all of this is the fact that yesterday I had to cancel the first visit of the highly recommended physical therapist. He had scheduled two visits this week, and said that unless I otherwise advised him, he would keep tomorrow's appointment.

I hope Carol is up to it.

I hope he is as good as advertised.

I know both hopes are fingers in the dike protecting against the onslaught of Carol's disease.

We are now three days past the seizure and things seem to have settled back down into our regular patterns. I had lunch today with two of my usual group, one of the others now in Hawaii visiting his son, and the other off on some domestic errand. I left Carol in the care of a new aide substituting for the one on vacation this week. Because Carol slept most of the time after eating lunch, this aide looked for things to do, to the extent of cleaning windows inside and out.

Carol would surely have appreciated that.

Yesterday, the new therapist arrived. He is as advertised. We agreed on setting both unrealistic and more realistic goals. The former would be success in getting Carol back on her feet, confident enough perhaps, to again use a walker. The latter started at enabling her to sit up. That simple fact would facilitate my dealing with her change of clothes. More ambitious progress would extend that sitting up to a stand and sit transfer into the transport chair so that I would be able to wheel her to the table and maybe even outside, although that latter would involve figuring out how to navigate steps.

Besides setting these goals, we also discussed strategy of treatment. I was delighted to discover that he believed in going very slowly. The implementation of that strategy during this first visit centered on his establishing a level of rapport through a lot of conversation. He did a little bit of range of motion exercises, but mostly talked. Every once in a while, I would add a comment to his patter; just to keep it moving along.

All in all, a very good start.

I will end this writing session on that happy note, for if I continue I will no doubt feel compelled to state the usual cautions.

They can wait.

Good Friday night and also the first night of Passover. Carol is asleep, and I am snatching a little writing time away from watching the Dodgers game streaming on MLB Network. This will be a short session, perhaps developed at greater length over the weekend.

If we were still in New York, or if Carol were still well here in Michigan, I would nod my head toward my holiday by having matzohs and macaroons in the house and perhaps cook up a brisket for us and a couple of friends. That would be my substitute for a full-dress seder, which I haven't really experienced very often in my adult life. In New York, I don't recall us doing much more for Easter than getting some chocolate bunnies. Here in Michigan, we would usually be invited to a family celebration of the holiday, which when the kids were young on at least one occasion included an Easter egg hunt. More recently, as Carol's siblings would sometimes attend holiday activities at spouses' houses, we might go out with sister Jane and family to a buffet in town.

In short, neither of us were seriously invested in holiday celebrations, and left to our own devices would pay minimum attention to them.

So, I do not mind that we will pretty much ignore both holidays this weekend.

The game calls and will not be denied.

It is Sunday night approaching midnight. As expected, the holiday weekend passed quietly.

And that suits me.

I did a little book business and attended to a broken string on one of the blinds in the living room. I arranged for it to be picked up today by the woman from whom we bought these blinds years ago and who repairs them when necessary. She has family on the Peninsula and offered to pick up the blind today after visiting her relatives.

Winter decided to inform us that it was not done yet, offering some snow and wind on Saturday, followed by dropping temperatures today.

As I was thinking about what I could prepare for supper, the doorbell rang, and there stood Brad from next door, accompanied by Marty, two of my lunch companions. Brad had plastic containers in his hands, which he offered to me, saying that he was aware that it was Passover but Amy had prepared an Easter dinner for us.

Lovely people, dealing with their own problems but thinking of us. Brought a smile to my face and lifted my spirits.

Tuesday afternoon in the library. Lots of noisy chatter from some kids. Although it is again snowing, so far the predictions of a serious accumulation have not occurred. Roads are still clear. Snow is anticipated through the night.

We shall see.

An April snow is not particularly unusual hereabouts as the Facebook You Have a Memory on this Date reminds me by reposting images from years back showing the property around our house beneath a white blanket.

But this year, perhaps because of my circumstances, and because as well, Easter occurred two days ago on April 1, and not because income tax returns are due in twelve days, this snow, this year, puts me in mind of the provocative opening of T. S. Eliot's "The Wasteland," to wit, "April is the cruelest month...."

The poem is famously difficult, and this is not the place to even begin to suggest what that line leads into. Rather, I choose to look at it, more or less, out of its context to see what thoughts it leads me to consider.

First, this five-word declarative sentence just seems wrong. In the northern hemisphere where Eliot spent his entire life, April is the doorway to spring, to life returning from the dead cold of winter. It is no accident that Easter occurs in the beginning of spring. Its message of overcoming death would not play well in winter, but it fits the warming season. If vegetation can return from a dead-like state, then so can people who have died.

Of course, Eliot is well aware of these associations of religious belief with the annual cycle of seasons. What he is offering is a paradox, a seemingly contradictory, even absurd, statement, which nonetheless is true.

April can only be seen as cruel if its promise is not realized. Because we respond so strongly to the promise of revival, to the prospect of life returning with its usual vigor, we are that much more distressed when that doesn't happen.

The rest of the poem, built on this paradox, explores it with a wealth of erudite details drawing on anthropology and comparative literature, all of which make it the bane of any undergraduate student who is asked to deal with it.

I, though, will simply take that paradox and apply it to our experience with dementia.

First, complete Eliot's basic point. As the title of this poem suggests, he does not see the promised revival as arriving. Therefore, the hopeful expectation is not, and perhaps will not, be realized.

From there, it's an easy transference of terms. Just take every instance that seems to promise a positive outcome and equate it to the disappointment April presages.

Library now quiet, kids gone, but I have to get home.

Late at night. Wind howling. Forecast still predicting significant snow through the night and into the morning.

OK, let's make the connection.

During the course of this disease, this dementia, at least as I have been experiencing it, there have been numerous little aprils, the lowercase beginning letter being deliberate to indicate the difference with the month, and the quantity, many more than a mere one a year.

But the similarity with the poet's month remains. These little aprils raise expectations that are routinely disappointed. One would think that this repetition would by its very nature diminish the expectation that the promise will be realized.

But it doesn't any more than the annual arrival of April does not produce the hoped-for conquering of death that Eliot has in mind. True, the weather does warm, nature springs back to life, only to be followed by the inevitable death of winter. Again, of course, Eliot is probing for deeper meanings beyond seasonal cycles, but it is enough in this context to say that just as the hope of the season of April inevitably gives way to the winter, the hopes raised by the lowercase aprils during the course of the disease will yield to the reality of the dementia's crushing power.

What brings all of this into the present moment is the arrival of the most recent physical therapist who again raises the possibility that as good as he seems to be he will be able to make some progress toward modest goals, such as enabling Carol again to sit up, and perhaps even, with enough assistance, again sit comfortably in the transport chair.

It is not much, and it may not happen.

The lowercase april might well emulate its larger sibling.

But if nothing else it is better to live with realistic hopefulness than wallow in despair.

I'm sure Carol, if she were able, would agree.

Party of the First Part

According to the calendar, we are two weeks into spring. However, winter does not seem to be paying attention. The cold continues, as does the occasional snow. Several more inches are forecast for tomorrow.

It is approaching midnight, and since I have to rise fairly early tomorrow to accept the delivery of the repaired window blind, I don't want to stay up too much longer. Still, an idea wants to out itself onto the page.

My neighbor Wendy, who kept her husband home as he withered under the relentless attack of dementia, came to stay with Carol so I could go into town for my fasting blood test ahead of my annual checkup tomorrow.

On the way into town I was reminded of the last time Carol accompanied me into the lab for one of these occasions, which occur every four months. My memory blurs a little as I try to pin down which exact ride into town I am recalling, but I am guessing it was about a year and a half ago, before her disease had manifested itself so forcefully.

We had secured the handicap placard for the car, and Carol was still fairly mobile. Otherwise, she would not have been accompanying me to the lab.

However, this time we never did get there. As we drove, Carol became increasingly uncomfortable in the car. I did not know then, nor can I say for certain now, what exactly was distressing her. But distressed she was. Perhaps it was the motion as the car followed the up and down and winding road, the same road she had been traveling much of her life except for those years when she was not living on this peninsula.

As we neared town, her discomfort was so intense that I decided I could not contemplate taking her into the lab with me. I turned around and drove us back home. Once in the garage, I could not manage to get her out of the car. She was in a state of panic, or maybe, it was anger, but whatever it was, she was not going to cooperate. Finally, as I had done on other occasions when her behavior had gone beyond what I could handle, I called her brother Ward, who always seemed able to soothe and calm her.

Not this time. He could do no more than I and urged me to call 911.

I did. An ambulance came and she was taken, not happily, into the vehicle and I followed it to the hospital. There, predictably, we spent hours while tests were run, and the emergency room doctor consulted with both Carol's primary care physician and the neurologist she was also seeing. The result of the conferencing was the hypothesis that her behavior resulted from a new medication, I believe it was Namenda, that she had recently started. Since none of the tests indicated any other likely cause, this was a reasonable guess.

All during this time, she was very upset and disoriented. She insisted she wanted her husband and rejected the idea that I was, in fact, there. Eventually, she calmed down enough to be released, and I was able to take her home, pretty much without incident although she still was not comfortable sitting in the car.

I took her off that medication, and her behavior returned to its usual patterns.

Looking back with the clarity of hindsight, attributing this entire incident to the medication is perhaps overstated.

As in so many other ways, now clear to me but hiding their true identity at the time, this event was just dementia flexing its muscles.

Perhaps as a warning.

Or maybe a boast.

Saturday afternoon, an unusual writing time for me. But a couple of ideas are swirling around in my head and I want to snatch them, lay them out on the table, and see where they want to go. I am familiar with this kind of experience, of ideas seeming to rise up from some hidden factory deep in my brain whenever I am heavily involved in a writing project.

It will be lunchtime soon, so I will just get started dealing with this idea effusion, planning to pick it up later, perhaps even this afternoon, for what else am I going to do on another day when winter refuses to leave, offering temperatures going down into the teens, accompanied by occasional snow showers?

I don't know whether I am the party of the first part, or party of the second part in this journal. Sometimes it is Carol centric, others as Steve centric.

It is about both of us.

Sometimes the focus will swing one way, sometimes the other, but always it is about the bond between the two, that bond in the past, the present, and the future.

Tuesday night, squeezing in a little writing instead of watching a television documentary about how Hannibal crossed the Alps on elephants. I've heard that story, of course, but somehow it never registered in my mind as real. It was too spectacular, too long ago, seeming to exist in its own time and space, not the one I inhabit.

I've got that show set to be recorded along with the one following it on public television, that one about the famous Leopold and Loeb thrill killers in the 1920s. I have read about that case, and I recall Clarence Darrow tried to save the two young men from execution. I can't remember if he succeeded.

Though the shows will be available at my convenience, I find I record many more shows than I actually wind up watching. That is why I'll keep this writing session a little short, so I will be able to watch the thrill killer one when it actually is on.

I've been thinking about my relationship to Carol, using the terms party of the first part or party of the second part. Something is coming into focus, although I do not yet have a name for it. Instead, I can think of specifics that lead to some kind of understanding, and then perhaps a word to describe it.

The specific detail that jumps to mind is, admittedly, almost silly sounding when I look at it as others might. Nonetheless, it is a strong presence in my mind. It goes this way. Every day I cross the road twice, once in the morning to retrieve the newspaper, and then in the afternoon, to pick up our mail.

Each time I do so, I make sure I have my phone with me. Now, here comes the seemingly absurd part. I want to make sure that if I suddenly fall down from a heart attack, I will be able to dial 911. The possibility of a heart attack is not the absurd part. About twenty years ago, while we were still in New York, I had two coronary stents inserted to relieve blockages. I was asymptomatic at that time, but the stress test revealed the problem, and there certainly is abundant history of heart problems in my family, including my mother, two paternal uncles, one maternal aunt, and my father, although his problem arose when he was eighty-six while the others' lives were shortened by coronary disease.

Still, all that being true, why do I obsess about having my phone? Well, for one thing, houses north and south of us are some distance away, and there are none east and west where there is orchard on one side and undeveloped land on the other. Therefore, conceptually, I could lie on the ground unseen for some time. On the other hand, if I had landed on the road a car driver might see me, or more likely ride over me, in which case, the phone would do me no good.

Writing this out demonstrates how ridiculous these ideas are. But what is not ridiculous is the stimulus for these thoughts.

My bed- and dementia-ridden wife would not know what

had happened to me nor would she be able to respond to it if somehow she were made aware of my lying outside somewhere.

It is necessary to point out that my concern is not primarily my own safety.

Rather it is I have to keep myself alive.

For Carol.

Wednesday evening after a quiet day at home. Spent an inordinate amount of time revisiting family history on my mother's side, prompted by shortcuts on my desktop to census documents, which in turn reminded me that grandson Peter wanted to know my mother's maiden name for his own family research project. I sent links to the documents to him, care of his mother Kerri, but then jotted down what I remembered about that side of the family, and when I could not recall a detail, I dug out a folder that contained the information.

All of which was a useful distraction on a day when not much else was going on.

Tomorrow, I have an appointment with the dermatologist to check out precancerous cells on my scalp.

Which leads into what I was writing about last session.

Namely, how my thoughts concerning my own mortality are now inextricably bound up in my self-defined role as Carol's caregiver.

Ordinarily, I don't dwell on my demise. And I wouldn't be doing so now except for the responsibility I feel for Carol. I confess I am concerned about how she would fare without me. Somebody would have to take over.

But who?

Our daughter now lives in Minnesota and has not yet established herself solidly on her career path as a programmer. She is getting closer to that goal, but it is not at all certain where she will wind up living. Probably not here because the job she seeks is likely not going to fortuitously turn up where the main industries are farming, tourism, and medical care of an aging population.

Of course, there are Carol's siblings, but frankly I don't see any of them stepping forward. At the moment, they are still involved with their mother, now living in a care facility herself, and otherwise they seem to be settled into their own concerns.

Which do not seem to include their sister in any meaningful way.

So, I think my concerns are just realistic.

Which leads to the exaggerated, somewhat comical concern of making sure I have my phone with me so I can call 911 should I find myself disabled on the road on the way back from the mailbox.

Somehow in my imagination, the disabling incident always occurs on my way back.

Perhaps it is my fiction writer's flair for the melodramatic.

Struck down steps away from his ailing wife. Mail strewn across the road.

A letter from his publisher in one hand, the other reaching for his phone.

Which he left in the house.

Party of the Second Part

As I write about us, I have proposed myself as the party of the first part and Carol, of course, is the party of the second part although I admit she would no doubt bridle at the second billing.

In any event, I will now focus quite directly on her through the lens of her journals.

Sunday night, the end of a weather-dominated weekend wherein a raging snowstorm, perhaps unaware of, or indifferent to, the calendar showing us to be in the middle of April, arrived Friday and still hasn't found the door out. Saturday morning I removed a foot of snow, some of it accumulated into drifts nearly twice that height. This morning more snow fell and drifted, but removing it proved much harder because it was mixed with ice. I decided to skip my usual Sunday morning visit to the local market even though I had cleared the driveway well enough to get the car out. With all the ice and snow, it just seemed a better idea to stay in the house. I am a creature of habit, and so it was with great reluctance I came to this decision. No doubt, in part, I was influenced by my concerns previously expressed about making sure as best I can that I keep myself safe.

My mind does flash to the end of Malamud's The Assistant wherein Morris Bober, who I believe is younger than I, dies of pneumonia after shoveling an early spring snow.

As to my health, I was glad to receive the dermatologist's judgment that the spots on my head, at this point, were not dangerous. As a precaution she sprayed them with liquid oxygen to freeze them off and had me schedule a follow-up appointment in a couple of months.

One less thing to worry about.

Because dealing with the weather these past few days has sapped my energy and eaten up my time, I am only now getting back into a writing rhythm. In so doing, I have extended these introductory, here and now, remarks and now feel I should think about sleep. If I were living alone, I probably would be indifferent to the clock, maybe even as I almost always did, read in bed for half an hour or so, but Carol will rise when she does, and her needs will call to me, sometimes with serious insistence.

So, I will, as I sometimes do, just begin what I intend to explore in my next session with my laptop.

In considering Carol's journals, and in reviewing the journals themselves, a couple of ideas emerge.

Those journals primarily cover 2005–2006. One of them then continues briefly seven years later not long before Carol's bout with breast cancer.

In them, I noticed the almost frenetic energy with which Carol was trying to shape her fiction, first her stories, and then a possible novel, or nonfiction book, and finally at the end of the period covered by the journals, a reasonable compromise moving from short stories to book length publication by marketing her stories as a collection.

I think I now understand two factors, which unnoticed at the time explain this intense energy.

The first belies an assertion that I had made that the years in question covered by her journal entries were unremarkable.

Not so.

They were remarkable in one most significant way: our daughter left for college and we became, although I never thought in these terms, empty nesters.

I don't know if Carol saw herself as the mother bird watching her fledgling take flight, but it seems abundantly plausible that she consciously or not was profoundly influenced by our daughter's leaving.

In danger of getting too caught up with this line of thought, which would result in inadequate sleep for me, and thus lead to a difficult day, when the weather, according to a recent forecast, promises to continue unpleasant.

Monday night. Just short of a month into spring and yet another day of snow dumping four or five inches. Snow-blower acting like it just has had enough. Tosses the snow but barely moves. I had to supply the muscle to get it up and down the driveway. Not a very good idea, but I do get stubborn. As I was straining, I worried about Carol in her bed, but continued anyway.

Dealing with the weather yet again has left me too tired to write tonight. Hope to pick it up tomorrow although it is my shopping day.

Tuesday night. Another six to eight inches of snow. Neighbor Rocco on his riding snowblower cleared the driveway in time to provide access for the nurse practitioner, then the aide, who came with a trainee, and finally, for me to get out and to the stores.

Carol never indicated how hard it was for her to deal with our daughter's leaving. Perhaps she herself was not aware. Outwardly, she was delighted. She had invested so much time and emotional energy in enabling Danielle to overcome her Asperger's sufficiently to let her native intelligence carry her through school and into college.

And there probably was a certain amount of relief for Carol as well. Satisfaction, too, of a job well done.

Later, when Danielle had graduated and gotten her first job in Cleveland, we refitted her bedroom as an office for Carol. In it, she could devote herself much more fully to her writing career.

That explains part of the stimulus for that frenetic energy evident in the journals. But there is that second factor, which this late I have come to believe was just as important.

In 2005, the year Carol starts her journal writing, my novel *Murder On Old Mission* came out. I now believe its arrival amplified Carol's writing ambition.

Of course, one reason I am late to this realization is that I had already published five novels during the time we lived together. The publication, therefore, of another novel from that perspective does not appear particularly significant.

But I now think it was.

For several reasons.

First, Carol's own career seems to have stalled after significant early success with her short stories. One of them, "Dancing Feather Light," appearing in the *South Dakota Review*, attracted the attention of a well-known New York agent, who contacted her to see if she could send him a novel. Stories are all well and good, but they rarely generate anything like serious money. Novels can. Others of her stories were recognized with prizes.

However, in 2005 those successes were beginning, I suppose, to look like they were in the rear-view mirror. Without checking dates, I am fairly confident in saying they all predated our move to Michigan. And the prospect of a novel dangled by the agent's query no doubt motivated her to try the longer form.

Then my novel came out, based on a suggestion from Carol's father, and set on this very peninsula on which she had grown up and on which we now lived. The book did well locally, receiving critical praise. Carol, no doubt, was happy for me. I do remember her saying early on in our relationship how delighted she was to have fallen in love with another writer.

Still, putting all this together, I now see that she so much wanted to get her own career back in gear but was finding it so difficult. There was her ADD, which her journals make clear she always battled. In fact, there is a brief note written in a large hand in her journal that "He," meaning yours truly, "will never understand my ADD."

There was the vacuum created by our daughter's moving out on her own, and then there was my very local, but still intense, success rooted in her turf. I can even imagine that had that 2005 book been set in my hometown of Brooklyn, as two of my earlier novels had been, it would not have moved Carol as much to get her own book out.

Now, with the clichéd wisdom of hindsight, I can see how hard Carol worked in those years to get her own book out. My guess, knowing the strength of her ambition and her stubbornness, she would eventually have succeeded. She had overcome so much, her natural shyness by getting her JD, her small town rural consciousness by immersing herself in New York, her acrophobia by willing herself to travel by plane, all of those obstacles unable to block her on her way to wherever she chose to go, convince me she would have gotten her first book out, and then there would have been others.

Had not first cancer, and dementia intervened. The cancer alone would only have slowed her down. But the dementia, striking at her cognitive abilities, was too big a barrier.

One last, sad note on this topic, at the end of the journal that continued into 2013, I observe that her wonderful handwriting was beginning to deteriorate, just a little.

Another very early, unnoticed, sign, not visible to me until a few days ago, of the beginning of where we now are.

New parents, ca. 1990. >>>

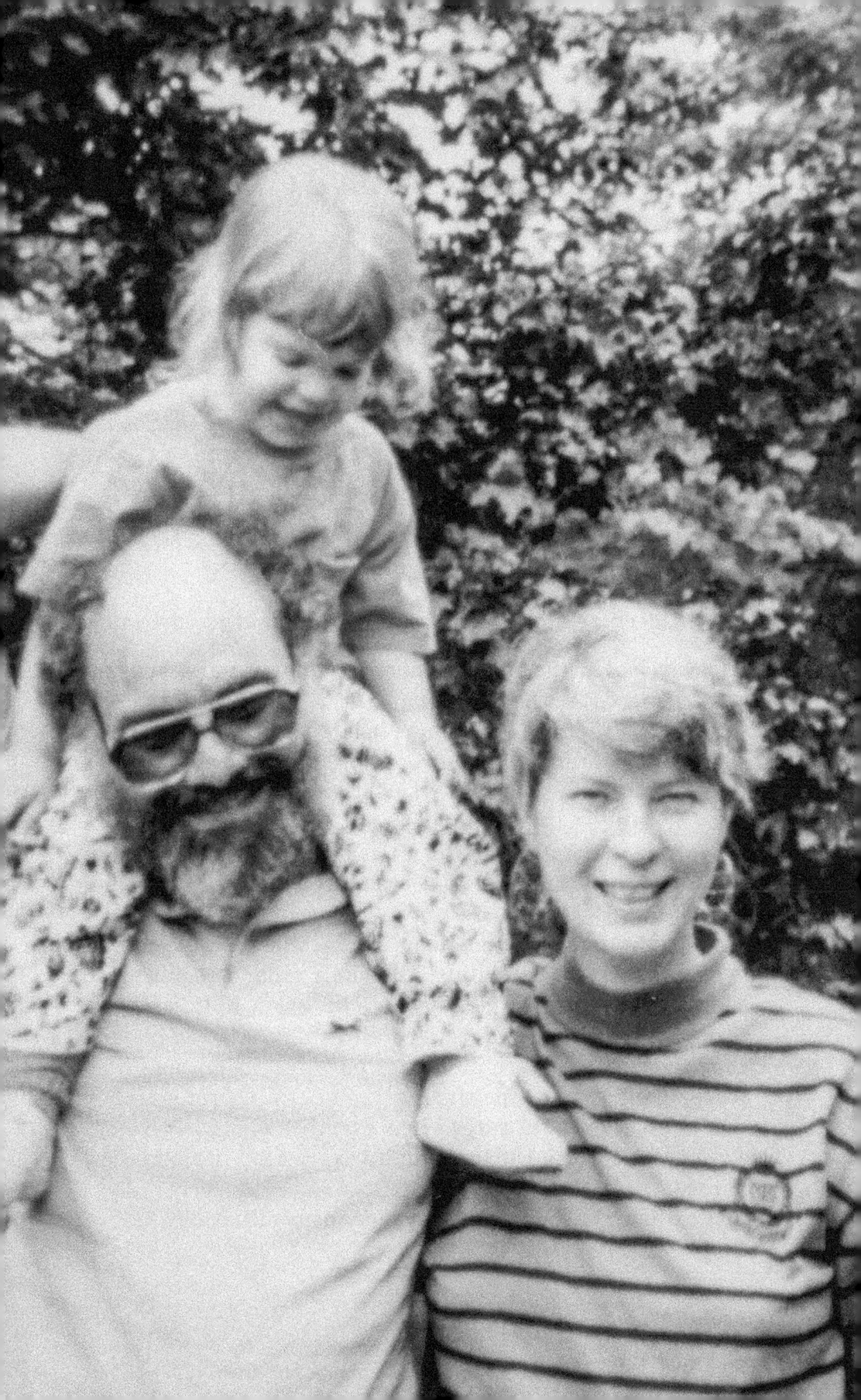

Hope Rides in on a Chair

Sunday afternoon. Spring has finally arrived. Swaths of browned grass emerging from beneath the snow on the margins of the lawn. Still significant piles of snow in other places, but the process has started.

Solitary bicyclists riding up and down Center Road. Soon, they will gather into packs and spill over into the roadway, asserting their right to the same road as the cars. On this twisty, hilly state highway, not always a sensible choice, particularly when there are ample shoulders to accommodate bicyclists even two abreast.

Carol sleeping, classical music from WSHU in my earbuds.

The arrival of the sun and warming temperatures suggest an upswing after the very long winter. Along with the seasonal shift, there is a tenuous reason, shadowed by a great deal of uncertainty, that our lives might improve.

Kyle Hamilton, the new physical therapist, messaged me a week or so ago with pictures of a tilt wheelchair. In truth, I did not know what it was until I asked him. I could see that it was a wheelchair, but there wasn't enough detail beyond that.

It turns out that, as the name suggests, this wheelchair's hydraulic system can adjust the chair from a reclining to a sitting up position and anywhere between. Kyle, who saw this particular item advertised on Craig's List, explained that because Medicare no longer pays for them, manufacturers have stopped producing them, and therefore, they are, in his words, "as rare as hen's teeth."

I appreciate both the fact and its expression in that hoary phrase.

But what, I asked, is its relevance to my situation?

It will be a boon to Carol, he declares, get her out of the bed, reduce the threat of pressure sores from lying on her back, enable me to wheel her about the house, even take her to the outside.

All well and good, I respond, but do you really think we will be able to get her into it, or to use your jargon, enable transfer?

Having worked with her a couple of times, and after extensive conversations with me, he believes this improvement might be in reach.

He came to this conclusion not only from his own observation, but also by factoring in my insistent emphasis on Carol's paralyzing fear of falling. If we can tamp down that fear, he thinks, she might regain the confidence to first sit up, then stand up, and if she does those things, she can then be helped out of the bed to a standing position and then to sit in the chair.

He provided what seems to my layperson's mind a very logical analysis. Having learned from me that Carol long ago was acrophobic, and that only by an exercise of her formidable will did she overcome that fear sufficient to enable us to fly, he concluded that her dementia had robbed her of her executive cognitive functions, so that the fear, which he describes as primitive, reemerged with nothing to counteract it now.

Therefore, if we can diminish that fear there is a reasonable chance, as years ago she was able to work through it and get on a plane, that perhaps now she can reach the more modest goal of getting out of bed and into this marvelous chair.

I take due note of all the qualifiers.

Nothing is certain.

But certainly, worth a try.

What we need is something to tamp down the fear.

His answer is buspirone, an anxiety-reducing medicine that he says he has had good success using with other patients.

He provided video evidence showing an elderly man pushing backwards as he is encouraged to stand.

Just as Carol now does.

But later, standing, and even walking.

The result of a regimen of buspirone.

Carol is now on it. He noticed her being more cooperative during his last session as he worked her with stretching exercises.

We shall see.

I have noticed a troublesome increase in drowsiness and some loss of appetite. I am told that these conditions might well be the body adjusting to the new medicine. It is very hard to isolate causes, to divide those resulting from the meds, and those the product of the disease itself.

The situation will have to be, and will be, monitored.

I know, too well, how extraordinary it would be to achieve this reversal.

I did ask Kyle for the width of the chair so I could see if it would, in fact, fit through the doorways in this old farmhouse.

It will.

Fragile hope is growing along with the warming sun.

As if in counterpoint, from outside comes the roar of motor-cycles, indifferent to all those still inside.

Tuesday night after an ordinary day of my shopping while the aide gave Carol a full bed bath.

I continue to monitor Carol's drowsiness and diminished appetite, trying to determine how much of these two conditions result from the progression of the disease on the one hand, and her body's getting used to the new med on the other. Today, she ate a full breakfast, but the aide said she was not interested in lunch. She was sleeping when I came home, but when she got up expressed interest in supper and finished off the frozen lasagna I always serve her on shopping days.

I don't cook on shopping days.

Yesterday, Kyle started his visit by measuring doorways to confirm what I had already told him in response to his concern, namely that the tilt wheelchair he wants me to buy will pass through these openings.

It will.

He worked very hard to take a step toward providing a solid reason for obtaining this wheelchair. He assures me that the price is a bargain, that years ago when his family got such a device for his quadriplegic father, it cost, literally, thousands more.

We agree that although the price is a steal, the main question is whether it will be of use to Carol.

Kyle was reasonably sure when he first proposed my getting it.

After today's session, he was more convinced, as was I.

Because with great skill, determination, and patience, he got Carol to sit up on the side of the bed, and then bodily lifted her into our travel chair. She was not at all happy being made to sit up and resisted strongly his first several attempts.

He persisted, offering self-effacing chatter, attempting to bribe her with offers of money if she would cooperate, and finally obtained sufficient cooperation from her to get her into the travel chair where she sat, more or less comfortably for perhaps ten minutes.

Then she did what she has always done when in that chair, and that is to slouch and start to slide off.

With my help, we righted her once, but when after a few minutes she started again to slide, we decided enough had been accomplished for one day, and Kyle hoisted her back onto the bed, where after a few moments she appeared to be again comfortable.

Lying flat on her back.

Still, progress had been made, sufficient to feed a small stirring of hope in tune, for the moment, with the promise of spring settling in outside our door where I see the daffodils, free of their snow blanket, raise their heads to the sun.

Wednesday night. Carol and dog sleeping. I am starting this writing session a little earlier than usual because I am tired. It's been an eventful day.

Or more precisely, it was a very quiet day until Kyle arrived at about six o'clock.

As he did last time, Kyle chatted, joked, and prodded Carol into some very positive results. He managed to have her sit up on the side of the bed two or three times. She offered strong resistance the first time, but after he let her rest for a while, the next times went more smoothly. She sat quietly with him at her side. He worked the bed's controls so that both the head and the foot of the bed rose forming a kind of valley where she sat with cushions placed behind her to support her back, and her feet over the side and reaching the floor.

All of this took some time, and I didn't think he was going to attempt much more.

But he did.

He wheeled the transport chair over next to the bed. He sat in it and pulled the seat belt around himself, trying to guess at a setting that would fit Carol. Then, having asked me to stand behind the chair to steady it, he placed one arm under Carol's legs at the back of her knees, and the other around her upper back and lifted her into the chair.

He secured her with the belt. I remained behind the chair, stroking her cheek, assuring her she was quite okay.

And she was.

And she sat.

Kyle wasn't done.

He wheeled her over to the dining room table where I removed a chair from the head of the table to make space for the transport chair. For reasons we have not yet determined, she always looks either straight ahead or to the left.

Kyle had me sit where I would be in her line of vision on the left and took the chair on the other side.

There were three fortune cookies on the table from Monday night's Chinese takeout. I offered Carol one, read her fortune, which had something to say about behind every able man was another able man, and I played with the gender designation a bit. Carol happily ate the cookie.

I was quite pleased that she did because her appetite has diminished on buspirone and Keppra which she takes to prevent another seizure.

Then Kyle wheeled her back to the bed and lifted her into it.

Carol did not always accept these transfers without expressing her unhappiness in a voice that hit some loud, high notes. Other times, she was quiet and accepting.

All in all, quite a productive hour.

I believe Kyle pushed faster than I thought he would, although remaining careful not to stress Carol, because he plans to close the deal on the tilt wheelchair. Convinced now that it will work for Carol, he will pick it up from Cadillac on Sunday, and bring it here.

He will need to customize it to conform to the dimensions of Carol's frame.

I did not know that was involved, but he says it is and he has done it before, just a little deconstruction and reconstruction.

He remains confident that, given the progress he has made, we will reach a point where I alone can get Carol into and out of the chair. She will spend her days in it instead of the bed. She will eat at the table, and perhaps even, with the help of some ramps, be wheeled outside.

Where she can see the daffodils close-up.

And perhaps with some kind of implement do a little gardening.

Grandiose?

Perhaps.

But why not aim high and see how close we can get?

The Chair

Friday afternoon in the main library in town. This is a lovely building constructed some twenty years ago, and it is bustling in a quiet kind of way, with a variety of patrons. That variety is the primary reason I drove the extra ten or so miles past the small community branch to which I usually go.

Sitting across from me is a Native American man, who judging by the plastic trash bag tied to his suitcase, is homeless. A young woman who had been working industriously at a neighboring table just packed up her things, including two computers, walked over to this fellow, and handed him a couple of bills, two twenties, I think. He demurred, saying he was fine.

But he took the money.

He mostly sits, eyes sometimes closed, but also takes out his phone every once in a while. Perhaps he is expecting a message.

It is good to get out of my bubble and see how the rest of the world is getting on.

He has moved to the table vacated by the young woman. Apparently on it there is a port for charging a phone, as he has plugged his into it.

A colleague years ago told me that he believed I am a people watcher.

Of course, I am. That is why I write fiction. Perhaps this man, and that woman, and their brief interaction will wind up in a story.

Carol is having a pretty good day. She ate her breakfast

with some enthusiasm and seems less drowsy. Last night, as well, she finished off her supper.

Perhaps her body is adjusting to the new meds. If so, I am relieved. I don't know much about precisely how her disease wreaks its damage, but I am on the lookout for lack of energy and appetite.

The Native American man has just walked over to talk to a man at another table. They seem to know each other.

There is an obvious train whistle coming through this building's windows. The depot building for the Pere Marquette train line is nearby. Google tells me that building, dating from 1927, now houses a microbrewery establishment. The train whistles emanate from freight trains.

And I just heard another train whistle.

Native American man now hunched over his phone.

I have clearly been distracted. But I am not at all unhappy. In fact, I am delighted to have broken out of my isolated little caregiver's world. Even more so to learn something new about this town, after living for sixteen years fifteen miles up the road from it.

These distractions, however, have taken me away from writing about what will be happening on Sunday when Kyle arrives with the tilt wheelchair and we start the process that might result in a dramatic change to that world in which Carol and I have been living.

Monday night after an exhausting but quite productive day. It is approaching midnight, and I have just enough energy to write what will amount to a head note to be developed at the next opportunity, perhaps tomorrow night.

So with that limited objective in mind, I can state that this day, the last in April, was the best in a long time. First, Carol ate three good meals, the last being most notable. Second, I managed to get to town to deal with my own medical problem, a highly irritating infection in my left eye. Third, Kyle devoted his session to making an adjustment to the chair he had dropped off yesterday. Fourth, he got Carol into the chair, and wheeled her out onto the deck. Fifth, Ward, Carol's younger brother and father of Ryan, expressed his desire to stop by this evening. Sixth, he joined us, Carol and me, and Ryan for dinner, with Carol in her new chair sitting at the table with us. And seventh, I managed, with Ryan and Ward standing by, to lift Carol out of the chair and back onto the bed.

All of this is noteworthy. I will decide how to shape it when next I sit down to write.

Tuesday night. Time to pick up the thread where I dropped it.

Before breakfast I debated with myself whether I should transfer Carol to the tilt chair. I had performed the reverse action last night, transferring her into the bed while I had help available if needed.

This morning I would be on my own. Another complication was the fact that today's aide who would be giving Carol a bed bath would be arriving in a few hours, after breakfast. Perhaps, I thought, I should take the simpler route and wait until I returned from town later and then do the transfer while the aide was still here.

I asked Carol if she wanted to get back in the chair, like last night, and eat her breakfast in the kitchen. To my surprise, she said she did.

I decided to take the plunge.

My first task was to reassemble the pieces of the chair that I had removed last night so as to eliminate anything that would be in the way of moving her into the bed. Those pieces included both leg rests and the left arm rest. With these pieces off when I positioned the chair next to the bed, there was nothing in the way.

They were now lying on the unused leg of the sofa. I wanted to be sure that once she was in the chair, I would be able to put the pieces back on.

It took a little time to remember what went where and how. Fortunately, my memory was good enough so that with only a couple of snags, I was able to get everything back where it belonged.

Then I took them off and moved the chair into position next to the bed. I made sure to tell Carol what I was about to do.

I put her shoes on so that if during the transfer process she put some weight on her feet, the shoes would provide traction on our slippery wood floor. Then, modeling my actions on what I had seen Kyle do, I first swiveled Carol on the bed so her feet were over the side and touching the floor. I then slipped my arms underneath her armpits and wrapped them around her as in an embrace. I took a breath and lifted her up.

I'm not sure if her feet ever did hit the floor. What I am sure of is that I was able to swing her into the chair.

She gave one little verbal complaint, but then settled in. I put the various pieces back on, found the gate belt and secured it around her waist.

And very happily wheeled her into the kitchen next to the table. There she sat while I fixed her breakfast. She was alert and ate without much hesitation. After she was done, I fed the dog, let her out, walked across the road to get my newspaper, and then prepared my breakfast.

Carol seemed to be getting drowsy, so I wheeled her back into the living room, tilted the chair back, and she was soon asleep.

The aide arrived, accompanied by a trainee. I asked the aide if she was familiar with this kind of chair. She said, no, but she knew about wheelchairs. I showed her how I had prepared the chair for transfer. And then left to do my shopping.

When I returned later, Carol was in the chair. The aide said that it had taken the two of them to get Carol onto the bed for her bath, and then off and back into the chair. Carol, they said, had stiffened her back, so that they had to struggle to complete the transfer.

That is not surprising. All of this was new. And she had just had the bed bath, which she is not always happy about.

I suggested, as Kyle had indicated to me, that through repetition Carol might become more comfortable with the transfer process.

We had supper at the kitchen table, and without too much stress, but not as smoothly as I would have liked, I got Carol back into bed, where she is now sleeping.

I expect with Kyle's help I will refine my transfer process. The whole idea is to avoid my having to bear her weight.

All of this detail probably obscures the significance of what has been accomplished these past couple of days.

Carol has been out of that bed for the first time in months. She has eaten at the table. She seems somewhat energized.

I know too well not to start thinking ahead. This is all very well and good. Perhaps it augurs a stay in the inevitable decline.

I will permit myself just a sliver of a hope that it might be a little better than that.

That hope, like a sliver of sunlight through darkening clouds, is enough to brighten our lives, at least for a little while.

A Useful Fiction and Real Progress

Friday afternoon. In the main branch of the library, look-
ing out of the window at the Boardman Lake, out of which
flows the Boardman River, which, in turn, empties into
Grand Traverse Bay a mile or two from here. I can see the
old railroad tracks on a swath of green. Beyond that is a
small parking area bordering the lake.

Altogether a charming view. I cannot imagine a better
spot, redolent of history and natural beauty, on which to
plant a library.

I am getting more practiced transferring Carol from bed
to chair and back. She accepts these movements without
too much opposition although she still exhibits moments of
panic as she is between the two.

When I came home from my shopping on Tuesday, the aide
told me that she had great difficulty effecting this transfer and that it took her and the trainee who was with her
that day to get the job done. That tells me that Carol was
offering significant resistance because this aide is both
physically and professionally competent. She is the one who
gives Carol her weekly bed bath. In fact, she was teaching
the trainee how to execute that task.

Perhaps it was all more than Carol was in the mood to
accept. And in spite of her dementia, Carol's base personality remains very much in evidence, and that base has an
ample store of toughness and independence.

The bad taste from that afternoon seemed to have spilled
over to Kyle's session the next day when even his best banter
and blandishment could not elicit much cooperation. He
came with the ambitious expectation to move to the next
step, which was to work with Carol so that she would handle
a stand and sit transfer, whereby she would get off the bed

into a standing position, turn ninety degrees and sit down into the chair.

He could not get Carol into a sitting position, which would be the precursor to getting her feet over the side of the bed.

She was having none of it.

Kyle did not push the issue. That is one of his finest attributes as a therapist. He knows when to stop, something previous therapists did not seem to understand. He said he did not want his voice associated with what seemed to be Carol's memory from the day before.

So, he just stopped and said he would try again on his next visit.

My respite time is drawing to a close. I will try to resume and round this off tonight or tomorrow.

Sunday night. As per usual watched Masterpiece *alone in the TV room. The dog remained in the living room.*

Kyle will be here tomorrow evening no doubt to try again to condition Carol into a stand and sit routine.

Whether or whenever he is successful, the presence of the chair has already had a positive effect. For the most part, Carol and I are eating together at the table, either in the kitchen or the dining room.

Well, to be more accurate, we sit together, but usually I help Carol eat first, and then I turn to my own food. But the point, as small as it might seem, is that I have been able to move past the mealtime fiction I have been observing particularly for supper when I set two plates on the dining room table. Then, I have been bringing over the meal in service plates, and while sitting in Carol's chair, fill up her plate with as much food as I think she will eat. Having done that, I carry the plate over to her bed and serve her meal to her there.

For all these months, I have been doing supper this way, always setting the supper table for two.

But now when I do that, I bring Carol over in her new chair, and we do sit side by side at the table.

In the mornings, I had been eating my breakfast alone after taking Carol hers. Now, we eat together at the table in the kitchen.

Lunch is still not settled. Where Carol eats that meal depends upon how long she has been in the chair when lunchtime arrives. Sometimes, I may have decided it was time for her to be back in the bed. And, in any event, she seems to have less interest in lunch.

Thus, these details, as trivial as they are against the backdrop of the larger picture, serve to lift my spirits. On the one hand, I fully recognize that the course of her disease has not changed. On the other, notwithstanding that fact, they do manufacture another useful fiction that our lives sort of go on as before.

And those kinds of fictions are necessary.

Carol, on some level, seems to agree.

In the morning, I ask her if she wants to get into her chair and go to the kitchen for breakfast.

She says yes. If she hasn't articulated the word clearly, I ask again, and she repeats in a firmer voice.

The same holds for supper.

She tolerates my transfers into her chair with only minor upset.

Together, then, we both buy into this most useful fiction.

Tuesday morning. Carol in her chair, dozing after breakfast. I am snatching a little writing time before the aide comes and I go to town for weekly shopping. Want to set down two tracks to develop: progress Kyle is making, and entirely unrelated thoughts prompted by Saturday's Kentucky Derby. The two are joined only by time, but I don't want either to slip away.

After a nonproductive session last Wednesday, Kyle arrived yesterday with his usual optimism and forward-looking attitude. His plan, I thought at the time, was audacious, a big step from the slow, cautious approach he had been pursuing. I'm guessing, since we didn't talk about his thinking, that he saw last week's problem as an aberration, a bump on the road, and he had determined to erase any trace of it by moving boldly forward.

He had decided to see if he could get Carol to stand.

Perhaps because I had been successfully managing the transfer process into and out of the chair for the past five days, by carrying her, or because the dosage of buspirone had been increased a little, or some combination, Carol offered less resistance to his initial efforts to have her sit up next to him on the bed.

From that position, he tried to lift her into standing. That didn't go well, so he switched to another strategy. He transferred her to the chair. Doing so placed her immediately into a solid sitting position. He placed a walker in front of the chair and tried to get her to grasp its handles. He didn't have much luck with that maneuver, so again he switched to another approach.

He removed the walker, stood in front of her, and then several times he lifted her onto her feet. Later, he reported that although he was largely supporting her in these instances, to a certain extent she was putting weight on her feet.

A start toward her standing.

Perhaps with the support of the walker, or even on her own.

As a kind of reward, he wheeled her out the back door onto the deck to enjoy the early spring weather.

Somehow, he had observed in the rear of the garage a piece of wood that had been part of a platform bed I constructed many years ago. The piece had a flat surface and on one end a right-angle lip of two or three inches so that when laid on the ground it formed a kind of ramp.

I no longer remember how it fit on the bed. But it turned out to be just about the right size to provide the ramp he had previously envisioned as being helpful in easing the wheel-chair over the doorsill and onto the deck.

He marked the piece to indicate its proper width and indicated he would find a saw to cut it. I told him I could manage that and took the piece back into the garage where my ancient radial arm saw was available for the job.

It did most of the cut. But the lip raised it too high so that the bottom of the motor prevented the cut from being finished. I dug out my circular saw, finished the cut, and brought the piece back out to Kyle. He placed it against the outside of the doorway and nodded his satisfaction.

A little later, when we had sat outside for a while, he tested this makeshift ramp and judged it adequate. It is difficult to assess how much Carol processed what was going on.

But she did seem to enjoy the sun on her face.

We brought her back in, and I kept her in the chair, for Ryan was due shortly for his weekly visit. Kyle left, Ryan arrived, we chatted, and then I drove to town to pick up Chinese takeout. Carol ate with decent if not great appetite.

A most successful several hours.

It did not halt the progress of the disease.

But for the while it drove it back into the dark corner out of which it had risen.

I haven't forgotten that I want to deal with thoughts raised by the Kentucky Derby. Will get to it next.

Like Ocean Waves

After midnight Tuesday, up in my office on my desktop PC instead of in my chair with the laptop in the living room. Came upstairs to use my good toothbrush and decided to write a bit on this computer. Carol is comfortably asleep downstairs. I have a little concern being up here because her last seizure a couple of months ago was silent.

I won't stay up here too long. I just want to get this next section started and hope to be able to resume it tomorrow.

When I was growing up in Brooklyn, the Atlantic Ocean was a bus or subway trip of less than half an hour away. My buddies and I would just wear our suits beneath our jeans, roll a towel up into our back pocket and make our way by public transportation to Bay 8 of Brighton Beach, down the shore from Coney Island.

I spent one summer when I was thirteen with my family in a bungalow in Rockaway. Same ocean, just some miles east.

In short, I became very familiar with the ocean. In particular, I learned, as a matter of necessity, how to handle the ocean's waves. The one thing you did not want to do was get hit full force by a breaking wave. Those waves could easily knock you off your feet and under.

An unpleasant but not life-threatening situation.

You learned to either go over or under the wave depending upon where you were standing as it approached you. If you weren't too far out from shore where the waves would break, you would advance toward it and dive under it before it reached you and then surface on the other side. If you were further out where the wave was just starting to crest, your job was a little easier. You just went over the top of the cresting wave.

All of which is preface to the metaphor that has been sitting in my head since the Kentucky Derby on Saturday.

That's enough of a start. I can pick this up fairly easily when next I have the opportunity.

Friday afternoon in town in the library after a couple of errands.

Strange as it might sound, deciding whether or not to watch the Kentucky Derby this past Saturday caused me considerable stress. This seems like a decidedly unimportant television viewing decision.

But it wasn't.

Because it drew me back hard into the world Carol and I together had created and shared.

In the interest of historical accuracy, I will point out that I possess a picture of my young self, sitting uncomfortably on a horse somewhere on a family vacation trip. My dim memory of that event is that I could not convince the horse I was on to move in the proper direction.

In short, that brief, unsuccessful close-up experience with horse flesh did not do anything to change my indifference to horses and horse racing. That there are several racetracks in and around New York City including Belmont, home for the last of the Triple Crown of races, was a fact to which I paid no attention.

I do not know why horse racing didn't register in my consciousness since I enjoy competition in almost any form. It simply was not of interest to anyone in my family or among my friends or their families. It is true that members of my first wife's family, particularly her father, were serious followers of horse racing. But I was never invited to share that interest with them, nor do I think I would have cared to.

I had no objection to following, or betting on, the horses. I was just indifferent to them.

Until Carol changed that.

She grew up on a farm that still used workhorses as indicated by a picture of her father with two such animals. She had her own horse for a time and spent a year in a private high school in Pennsylvania, which featured, among other things, training in dressage, including jumping.

When she lived in New York, her life was filled with a whole list of new experiences and challenges, none of which involved horses. It is possible—my memory is uncertain—she might have taken me to a horse show somewhere on Long Island. I know we attended such an event. I just can't be sure where. Long Island, particularly in the upscale north shore communities, does have the kind of horse owning culture associated with old money. So, the show might have been there.

But when we moved to rural Michigan, we were in serious horse country. Our neighbor to the north until recently kept a couple of horses in a fenced area behind his house. The owners of the house we bought had a horse stabled in the building we converted into an office. Carol's brother and his wife had their own horses and also even now make their barn and pasture available to renters.

Respite time over. Will try to continue, perhaps tonight.

Monday night. Kyle had a tough session with Carol who was noncooperative. He cajoled her onto her feet several times.

Ironically, she awoke from a short nap after he left in a remarkably good mood, alert state of mind, and with a healthy appetite for the pizza we were sharing with Ryan.

Kind of a microcosm of the maddening ups and downs of this disease.

I'll try to pick up the thread I dropped a couple of days ago.

All of my ruminating about horses is the context for my

dealing with the Kentucky Derby. Doing so reminds me, if such is necessary, of another indication of Carol's love of horse racing, so here it is.

Some years ago, in fact I believe not too long after we moved here, Carol took herself off to a writers' retreat. Three details remain in my memory. First, the Subaru dealer in town managed to mess up a routine service so that we deemed it unwise for Carol to take the car until the problem was resolved. That fact also helps date this incident within a year or two of our arrival here in 2002 when we were still relying on the dealer for service. Carol rented a car and went off.

I can't remember where exactly the retreat was, perhaps southern Ohio, but it was not far from Louisville. That is the second detail that is clear.

Which leads to the third. I flew down to join Carol, and together we went to Churchill Downs. It was off season. So, no race, but she thoroughly enjoyed walking about the grounds and building. I recall we also took a boat ride on the Ohio.

My musings about the Kentucky Derby take me back to the metaphor I had begun to develop built on my recollection of navigating ocean waves.

I simply could not make up my mind first whether to watch it. We always watched it together. Carol would study the horses being paraded before the race, and based on her familiarity with these animals, she would pick one to root for. I would choose based on a name or some other detail. On this occasion, I knew if we watched together, we would not talk about the horses, at least in any meaningful way.

Sitting in the green room with the television remote in my hand, I was paralyzed by an indecision that was rooted in the heavy wave of sadness that had rolled over me. It was the same kind of wave I experience regularly when I am forced to confront a reminder of what we used to share.

These waves can and do crop up without warning. There are hundreds of objects in this house that can be the occasion for one of them to arrive, uninvited and unwanted. I live among them. Most often they cause nothing. But then something, the silly sign in the upstairs bathroom announcing baths for five cents, or the laptop sitting idly on the desk we bought and set up in her now unused office, the nightgown hanging on a hook in the bedroom I enter only to retrieve my clothes, the salmon rub she insisted we buy still on the shelf in the cabinet in the kitchen, these and all the others I encounter every day every once in a while raise that wave of sadness that engulfs me.

Unlike the ocean waves, there is no learning how to dive under them or ride over the top of them. They will sweep over me.

But also unlike the ocean waves that smash you with tremendous force if you fail to implement one of the avoidance maneuvers, knocking you around and down, these waves of sadness instead are almost gentle, yes gentle, but not in a soothing way.

There is no physical beating.

Just the feeling of being enveloped in a gray mist, not black enough to lead to despair, but thick enough to create the physical sense of its cold embrace.

The moments pass.

But there will be another and then another, on and on, like the endless repetition of ocean waves against the shore.

Being a Caregiver

Tuesday night. Seattle-based jazz station streaming into my earbuds. Went into town for weekly shopping but with first stop at The UPS Store to send back an incorrectly ordered beard trimmer, one that did not have an adjustable length setting option, and while there also shipped a copy of my latest book to my old Fort Salonga friend, from whom I just received a stack of his films along with a novel. Also sent to Danielle a T-shirt decorated by grandson Brandon with images of cats, intended for Carol.

Sometimes a day is punctuated by everyday chores, such as arranging for a plumber to come fix a leaky kitchen faucet, or for Carol's hairdresser to come out to cut her hair. And sometimes, a chore is less ordinary, such as spending an hour on the phone, mostly on hold listening to all the wonderful services Michigan has to offer, while working my way to a person in the Secretary of State office who will authorize resending the forms necessary to provide Carol with a personal identification number, which can be used in lieu of her expired driver's license number for the next time I will file our income tax return. The form had apparently been sent in late March when I first became aware I would need one such down the road, but it never arrived.

Doing these mundane matters provides a small sense of accomplishment that is largely absent from my life these days. A very welcome glimmer of normalcy, however inconsequential, toward something a little better or as in the case of the personal identification number, necessary.

Before finishing for tonight, as I am tired, I will record one small but not insignificant moment from a couple of days ago and contrast it with a larger nonevent.

First the small one. I was working on my laptop in the

late morning researching markets for my writing. A Google search had brought up a useful list and I was exploring it for a while. Absorbed as I was in this task, I lost track of time. I happened to look up from the screen and saw Carol stirring in her bed. I glanced at the clock and saw we were already a little late for lunch.

I got up from my chair, walked over to Carol, and said lunch would be ready soon. I added an apology, saying, "I was just trying to make us rich and famous, and if not famous, I will take rich."

She offered a genuine laugh.

Once again, for that brief moment we were together in the here and now.

I knew it would not last, but I savored it.

Now the larger.

Mother's Day.

How to deal with it.

I could, of course, just ignore it. Carol would have no idea that it had arrived. This was the same kind of dilemma I faced with the Kentucky Derby the day before.

I had thought of buying a half dozen roses as I had for her birthday in January.

But somehow that idea didn't sit well with me. The best explanation I can offer for my discomfit was not so much that it would probably be a waste of money, but rather that it was a futile attempt to continue a fiction, to pretend that we were still living in a time of celebrating such holidays together that was most definitely gone.

I had mentioned this situation to the aide on Friday. She offered the very practical suggestion of cutting some of our daffodils, now in full bloom. I believe she is used to being quite frugal and so was probably drawn to this solution by it being cost free.

At first that idea did not appeal to me. But after a while I came to see it as a way of doing something I was comfortable with, probably because it was both fitting and new as I had never cut our own flowers to mark an occasion, although

I seem to recall bringing in some of our yellow roses last season.

Sunday morning I went out onto the front lawn to the daffodil bed and snipped off enough to fill a vase I had found in a closet. I placed the flowers on the kitchen table and wheeled Carol in.

I don't think she actually saw them although I placed them right in front of her eyes.

Yet, I am content that I had tried.

That afternoon our daughter called. Apparently, she had dealt with the issue from her perspective. She knew from her own experience that her mother could no longer respond to her as her mother. But she felt she should call.

So she did.

We had a long, warm, and useful conversation. I filled her in about how Kyle was working with Carol to get her on her feet, at least in a limited way, but mostly we talked about other things, how for the first time in sixteen years I actually happened to look out of the kitchen window when the flatbed truck arrived carrying the bees imported for the orchards across the road, how there was an article in the paper concerning a study of the feasibility of restoring passenger train service to our town, and other such.

It seemed right on Mother's Day to have a good conversation with our daughter, who after all, is the reason the holiday has any significance for us.

Last note. As I got into the flow of these ideas, I did not hear the music coming through my earbuds.

I hear it again now as it pauses to provide time for a news update concerning the unrest in Gaza.

The world will be heard, even here in the bubble that is Old Mission.

Thursday night. Carol asleep. I am tired. It seems I am always tired these days.

Which leads me to the idea that has been gestating in my

*head for several days. I'll see what it has to offer, or at
least start to do so.*

I remember hearing some time ago that people in my situation, that is caregivers, become just that, to the exclusion of what they had been before.

What does that mean?

Well, it opens the broader question of how do we think of ourselves, how do we define ourselves, how, in effect, would we answer the question, "What do you do?" That question is similar to, but more provocative than, "Who are you?"

The who are you question can be answered in a number of fact-based ways depending upon the circumstance in which it is asked. The question might simply require providing a name as in arriving for an appointment. Or perhaps its answer must place you in relationship to some other person, as at a social situation at which people who don't know each other, but do have some common purpose for being at the event, introduce themselves to each other, "Oh I work with so and so."

In contrast to those simple factual questions and answers, the "What do you do?" question demands self-definition. The answer that seems to spring to mind is to indicate what we do for a living. We define ourselves by our jobs. I am a lawyer, I teach, I own a restaurant, I am a housewife, or a house husband, I have a soybean farm. Whatever we spend most of our time doing, or perhaps better expressed, whatever we have to do.

To indicate the centrality of this kind of response, an answer such as "Oh, I am retired," usually elicits the follow-up, "Yes, but what did you used to do when, in fact, you had to do something?"

That's a start to looking at the point with which I began.

Do I now say I am a caregiver? And similar to a retired person, do I add but I used to be a college professor, or after that was no longer true, say I was a writer?

A start. Weariness is stopping the flow.

Sunday night. I'm looking across at the tilt wheelchair that has made such a difference. The leg rests and the left arm rest are off, removed to make transfer easier. I have WSHU streaming some nice music into my earbuds. Above the music I hear Carol's open-mouthed sleep breathing. On the floor to the right lies the sleeping dog offering an occasional doggy snore.

Let's see if I can pick up the thread and transition back to the question of what I am.

Doing the arithmetic of 24×7 tells me there are 168 hours in a week. For all of those hours, minus the nine of relief, or to be precise for 159 of those 168 hours, I am Carol's caregiver. That's a whole lot more than the traditional forty-hour workweek.

Of course, one could quibble and say, at the least subtract sleep time. I will give a qualified agreement and reduce 56 hours to account for sleep at eight hours per night.

That's a qualified concession because even when sleeping I am still on duty.

I sleep near Carol's hospital bed in part because I want still to be near her, to hear her breathing, or the occasional sleep talk she offers. But I stay close because I want to be sure insofar as I can that I will know if anything medically significant occurs so that I can respond to it.

All of this talk of numbers is natural to me. Focusing on quantifiable facts is one of the ways I mediate my interaction with the world, which makes more sense to me when numbers are overlaid onto the flow of events and perceptions.

But I am also making a point, however labored. Nothing I have ever done in my life up to this point demanded such a commitment of my time.

On that basis, if one identifies oneself by what one does, and if factored into that what one does element is the time spent doing it, I am a caregiver.

More than I ever was as a college professor or a writer. Of course, as a husband or a father, I was on in those roles every minute of every day. But just as clearly, I was doing other things at the same time.

Now as a caregiver, I am acutely aware that I always have one metaphorical eye on Carol whether I am attending to something outside, running off to the store, or as now, as she sleeps, sitting perhaps fifteen feet away writing on my laptop.

To put an exclamation point on the point, I can say that I do not spend much time in my office upstairs where I could work on my newer, more powerful, more comfortably situated desktop computer simply because I would feel I was neglecting my caregiving responsibilities.

I conclude, therefore, that what I am now, more than the writer I still try to be, or the retired professor with continued interest in his fields of expertise, more than anything else, I am a caregiver.

Not a job to which I had aspired, but one thrust upon me, and one I strive to do as well as I can for as long as I am able.

Music Hath Charms

Late Wednesday afternoon. Kyle will be here within the hour. We are nearing the end of Medicare-supported visits. Had a brief discussion last time about continuing his therapy on my dime. I don't know if that is practical. Carol has made such good progress under his care, but it is also possible we are nearing the ceiling of what he can accomplish.

The disease will win out in the end. The only question is where or when that end is.

I am not feeling perfectly well today. Even a restorative nap has not fully recharged my battery.

I will soldier on as I have always done. I have experienced very few debilitating illnesses that prevented me from going about my business. I had chicken pox as a young adult and that kept me home from my new teaching job for about a week. I have spent one night in the hospital when two coronary stents were inserted. There were probably a few other occasions that do not come to mind, but I have been remarkably durable, retiring after thirty-five years with most of my sick leave unused.

All of this is said in the context of my now self-defined identity of caregiver. More than at any other point in my life I cannot now afford to be sick to the point of becoming unable to function.

Kyle has just arrived. His arrival times are always approximate.

Saturday night. I have been too tired the past few days to attend to this writing. I think I might be dealing with a bug.

I've got my Simon and Garfunkel Pandora station streaming in my earbuds.

That is because a little while ago I played the CD of the duo's concert in Central Park.

I need to make two points about my choice to play this music.

The first is general concerning music, the second is particular to that concert.

Several days ago, as we were having breakfast, for some reason I took note of the small Sony radio sitting on the butcher block top of the wheeled cabinet that serves as an island in our kitchen. That radio has been there literally for years although we did not turn it on that often, just mostly to listen to *A Prairie Home Companion* while eating Saturday evening dinner.

But on this morning, I turned it on and fussed with the tuner until I found the classical music station from Interlochen. I listen to that station on my car radio, but for whatever reason not in the house.

I don't know what motivated me to turn it on that morning. I will say I am embarrassed I did not think to do so sooner. I knew, or at least was aware in a dim kind of way, that music is reported to penetrate the fog of dementia. In fact, one aide some time ago asked if she could play music, and if so, what did Carol like. I suggested blues, particularly of the Delta variety, and dug out a couple of CDs. I had plugged in an old boom box on the end table next to the sofa so I could play audiobooks for Carol. She listened with some interest to her favorite book, *To Kill A Mockingbird*, but others did not hold her attention.

We tried a blues CD. Carol did not listen, and we abandoned that idea.

However, her response to the classical music on the radio was positive. I saw her nodding her head to it and changing her facial expression to reflect changes in the music. Then, I remembered her father loved classical music. He had a large, old-fashioned stereo system set up in the dining room, and I was aware that he and Carol's mother attended concerts at Interlochen.

I don't know for a fact, but it is likely he played classical music on that stereo with some regularity. What I do know is that music was prominent in Carol's family. Her mother played the organ for her church for fifty years, Carol's sister plays violin for that same church, and others in the family play. Carol herself had years of piano instruction.

So it is not surprising that she responded to the somewhat tinny music coming from that little Sony radio.

I've been turning it on every morning since. And when we move into the living room, I tune to the same station on the boom box, and let it play all day.

Which takes us a step away from Simon and Garfunkel. Let's get back to them and their famous outdoor concert.

At dinnertime today, the programming on the radio turned to a nightly show that features a lot of analytical talk about the music being offered. Wanting to continue listening to music without the talk, I sorted through a pile of CDs next to the television.

Where I found the Simon and Garfunkel CD.

And now the particular reason for pulling it out of the stack instead of something classical like a Bach compilation that was also in the pile.

Carol had attended that concert.

That was in 1981 before she entered my life.

She often spoke of the experience, how far from the stage she and her companion were that they could not really see much, and how the music filled the park.

I asked if she would like to hear it.

"Yes," she said.

And she listened with head nods, foot wagging, smiles, and at least one laugh at one of the lyrics.

So, yes, music apparently does penetrate, does, perhaps, wake up some memories.

And we will continue to listen.

Past midnight of Memorial Day, the end of seventy-two hours of almost complete isolation, broken by one telephone call I initiated, one greeting to the owner and clerk at the market on my Sunday morning trip to pick up the *Times* and Carol's blueberry muffin, and two brief conversations with neighbor Brad. The first of those occurred in the street after I had picked up the mail and then strolled over to him where he was weed whacking some brush. I wanted to follow up on the suggestion I had offered concerning his getting in touch with our piano tuner to service the used instrument they had just obtained at a fundraiser. The second, brief, conversation with him during the weekend was occasioned by his stopping by with some food from a holiday barbecue at their church attended by a number of members of the historical society who sent their regards to me and Carol, a most welcome and unexpected visit. Even the telemarketers seem to have taken the weekend off. I initiated the one telephone call, phoning that same tuner to see if he could do our piano after Brad's. He called a couple of days later to say he would.

These arrangements concerning piano tuning lead naturally back to the reintroduction of music into our household. I now have the radios, one in the kitchen, the other in the living room, tuned to the Interlochen classical music station from morning to night.

I cannot be sure how consistently Carol listens, but sometimes it seems her head or her hand moves to the rhythms. In any event, her mood has been more even-keeled, and I attribute, however tentatively, that effect to the constant music.

The choice of classical music was a natural for me although, in truth, I like many genres. At the moment, KNKX, a jazz station from Seattle, is streaming into my earbuds. I listen to folk and to classic rock as well.

But classical music, I believe, is a better choice for Carol in her present condition. True, she used to love Motown and blues, as well as sharing my interests. However, without any research into the question, I am hypothesizing that the more complicated structure of classical music engages her brain more fully. That, plus the possibility of the music reawakening the auditory memories of the music she heard in her house growing up.

It would be foolish to suggest that Carol's listening to music can stay the progress of her disease. In spite of my generally optimistic attitude, I long ago gave up on the idea that anything less than divine intervention, which I confess is more than a little unlikely, would stop that progress.

All that can be done through medicine is trying to slow the inevitable deterioration, and as with Kyle's introduction of the tilt chair, improve the quality of our lives.

I don't know if the music now playing pretty much all day every day in our house will have the salutary effect of stimulating brain activity, and thus slow that deterioration.

But it certainly seems to have a positive impact on her mood.

And mine as well, as all my life I have listened to music whenever possible.

As William Congreve opined centuries ago, "Music hath charms to soothe a savage breast."

I don't know about the "savage breast"—often misquoted as "savage beast"—but its ability to charm in a variety of ways is palpable, a wonderful gift I will make a permanent resident of our household through these difficult times.

There is more to the relevance to our situation of the story of our piano and piano tuner. Will explore that in the next entry.

The Tale of the Piano

Thursday night. It's been a few days since I had the time and energy to write. It's not that late, but I don't feel particularly energetic. Today was active, beginning with the arrival of our piano tuner, followed almost immediately by my usual lunch out, this time with three of the four attending. A little rest when I came home, then supper preparation and into the evening.

Where last I left off, I was starting to talk about our piano. I'll pick up that thread.

Early in our marriage, our finances were, to put the matter gently, strained. I knew that Carol very much wanted a piano. She grew up with one in her house, her mother played, and she herself learned on it.

Not being able at that time to afford a piano, I instead bought a refrigerator magnet in the form of a grand as a promise that someday we would have an instrument, most likely not a grand, but a serviceable one that she could play. Eventually, we reached the point where our finances permitted the purchase of a used Musette, circa 1930. It offered a nice cabinet and matching bench, both featuring spindles and curved legs that somehow, at least to me, suggested something musical. And it produced decent sound.

Carol happily began reacquainting her fingers with the keyboard, working on, I recall, the "Moonlight Sonata" and Pachelbel's "Canon." I enjoyed listening to her play and to see how happy she was. We started lessons for our daughter.

The piano moved with us to Michigan. However, we did not hire a piano mover. Rather it came along with the rest of our belongings.

It did not survive the trip well.

Which leads to the particular piano tuner who arrived this morning to work on it.

Will pick this up next writing session. I think it is leading to something good.

Sunday night near midnight after a cool and rainy weekend. The weather cannot seem to make up its mind as we slide into June.

Where I left the piano story off, the instrument was installed in our new house awaiting to be tuned after its thousand-mile trip in the moving van. However, the tuner we hired declared that its soundboard was now cracked, and he could not tune it. Somehow, we managed to get it into the garage without having made a decision as to what to do with it.

Carol still wanted to play so we purchased an electronic piano. She never liked its sound although I enjoyed its ability to emulate various instruments, such as a harpsichord. That was not enough to keep it, so we gave it to Carol's sister.

I am compressing time to keep this moving along to its point, which I hope to reach before I forget what it is.

The piano from New York remained in the garage as we still neither came up with a plan for it nor felt particularly motivated to resolve the situation.

Until we needed that space in the garage.

Rather than figure out how to get rid of it, sell it, junk it somehow, whatever, I decided to revisit the question of whether it could be made to play in tune. To that end, I got in touch with local jazz pianist Jeff Haas and asked him who was the best available tuner. He recommended Brant Leonard, the tuner who came a few days ago to once again work on the piano.

He checked the piano in the garage, declared that, of course, he could tune it, and that it was just a question of getting the tension on the strings right. My recollection is that he then, by himself, moved the piano back to its original location in the house.

The piano, though, remains difficult to keep in tune,

primarily Brant says, because it sits in front of baseboard heating, which dries its wood every winter, loosening the pegs that hold the wires.

And there really is no other place in the house to which it can be moved.

Now, we are getting to the point of this story. Why did I, knowing how difficult the piano is to tune, and that I will not be able to keep it in tune over the winter without heroic, and at this time, ridiculously difficult, effort that involves sliding it out of its place every morning to fill up the humidifier that will keep it from drying out, and there is no doubt that I will find that chore too burdensome as I did last winter, and very likely will not do it—why in view of all that did I arrange once again for Brant to tune it on the same day he was tuning our neighbor's piano?

True, as long as he was coming out here, and since he charges travel time, we could split that part of his bill and both save a little money.

Which begs the question as to why I would want to tune it.

Carol of course is not going to play it.

I can play a little. I had a couple of years of indifferent lessons when I was about ten and much more interested in playing ball in the streets than practicing the piano. Still, I was always a good sight reader, as my teacher so many years ago declared while suggesting that I should try practicing between his lessons. With some effort I can still read as long as things don't get too complicated.

Getting too late to continue. Will try to finish this section tomorrow.

Tuesday night. Yesterday left me with no energy to write. The morning was ordinary enough, but then I had an appointment with the dermatologist in the early afternoon. She saw spots on my head that could have been new or the remnants of those she had removed some time ago. To be safe, she hit them with liquid nitrogen producing an effect very much akin to having an axe cleave your skull. I went home with a serious, lingering headache. Rested for a while, and then Kyle came for what was to be his last session. He said we had a few paid sessions left, and he thought it prudent to save them, particularly in light of his conclusion, to which I assented, that he had done what could be done to that point but other circumstances requiring his assistance might come up.

Back to the piano story. I have to add, as memory now insists, details in this evolving tale. Early on in dementia's attack on Carol, when we had no clear idea of what we were dealing with, when we both believed she was just suffering the aftereffects of chemo, which would wear off in time, she very much wanted to resume playing the piano. But she was having difficulty remembering how to find the right keys. That should have told us we were dealing with something quite serious, but we were ignorant, perhaps willfully so. She tried taking lessons. They didn't take very well. We stopped by a music store in town to get sheet music with which she could practice. She was thrilled, telling the owner of the shop that he had given her back something precious.

But he hadn't of course.

She still couldn't play.

With the piano again in tune thanks to Brant's wizardry, I sat at the keyboard from time to time seeing if I could learn to play Beethoven's "Gertrude's Dream Waltz." Which, I have learned, Beethoven probably did not write. No matter. It seemed within my limited reach.

I played it. Sort of. After a while I could read the notes and connect them to the keys, and I liked the sound.

I was kind of making music.

Carol could still hear when I hit a wrong note, and she would not hesitate to tell me.

I think I can now bring this meandering tale to a focus and to its point.

To do so, I have to answer the question already posed as to why I, at this late date, had this failing piano tuned yet one more time.

I believe the answer is composed of several threads, one of which is most important. First, I still want to work on Gertrude even though I have little time or energy for practice.

Second, and this is getting closer to the main thread, building on my interest in playing, even badly, I am doing something very specifically for myself. Carol is unaware. She no longer points out my wrong notes.

Third, as a corollary, the tuned piano represents a kind of transition, a bridge from the Carol past to the Steve future. It is both a reminder of Carol's attachment to the instrument she can no longer play and a glimpse at my life ahead.

When I will make decisions looking forward rather than back.

To be clear, I do not envision developing a serious interest in playing the piano. I may never tune this instrument again. And if I don't, I won't replace it either. That decision most likely will mark another step in the process.

The process of leaving behind the then, moving through the now, into the new future.

What is clear, though, is that I will carry our past into that future. That will be a mixture of necessary pain sweetened, I trust, by a little comfort.

Note: Since I drafted this post, the piano has again fallen out of tune—the E above middle C is seriously out. The piano is well on its way to becoming no more than a piece of furniture.

A stubborn reminder of what was, and an indicator, perhaps, of what will not be.

Kyle's World

Sunday evening. Carol is asleep. For the past four or five days I have been dealing with an old physical problem, one that has not really bothered me for some time. But it decided to remind me that it could still make my life miserable. I have been fearful of the return of this condition because in my present circumstances I cannot afford, Carol cannot afford, for me to be disabled.

I want to locate the problem in my back, but that may not be clinically accurate. The symptom of the problem, though, is clear enough, a shooting pain that accompanies the slightest movement, such as sitting down, or getting up, or walking, or picking up something, any such ordinary motion produces a jolt strong enough to make me grunt and stop whatever I am doing.

That nexus of that pain, as best I can locate it, is my lower right back and right hip area. It definitely does not feel like a joint issue. Rather I'd guess it is a soft tissue problem, a tendon or ligament stretched or strained.

This condition first introduced itself to me when I was in my thirties. Typically, it would slowly ease up over a couple of weeks. It was largely indifferent to rounds of physical therapy or treatments from chiropractors. Muscle relaxers didn't really help much, but a scotch and soda sometimes had some effect.

Now, however, I just have to grit my teeth and try to be careful although the motions that bring a stab of pain are so inconsequential there really is no way to avoid them altogether. Advil, which I don't recall ever trying in the past, seems to yield a few hours of relief.

All of this provides the immediate context for what follows, and which I will begin writing for as long as the Advil enables me to sit and hit the right keys on my laptop.

As usual I have been struck by how prescient Kyle had
been. His goal was to condition Carol to be able to stand
while supporting most, if not all, of her weight long enough
to then turn and sit down. This would be the essence of the
transfer from bed to wheelchair, and from wheelchair to
bed. The key was for her to cooperate in sitting up so that
her feet would reach the floor. She would have to be made
to overcome a primitive impulse to throw herself back. It
became clear that she would not do this by herself. But she
could be made to accept a hand behind her neck pulling her
into an erect sitting position.

That has been achieved. Sometimes she vocalizes her
unhappiness with being made to sit up this way, but most
often she accepts the pressure that achieves this movement.

The next step is to get her standing. The whole point of
this procedure is to avoid having to lift her up. Once she is
sitting, her feet must be on the floor. Sometimes she needs
encouragement, pressure on her thighs to get her legs down
and feet grounded. Then, with verbal encouragement, and
providing a little lift, she rises. Once on her feet, she might
need to be steadied, but she is bearing most of her weight.

When she is standing in a kind of embrace, my arms around
her, we do a little two-step shuffle to turn her around so that
she can sit again either on the side of the bed or the seat of
the wheelchair.

Throughout this procedure we have a medically necessary
physical intimacy that is both a mocking shadow of our marital physicality but also a present-time version that warms
my heart.

In any event, I have learned how to do this transfer fairly
well.

But now that my—I'll call it my back—is barking at me,
performing this process can be problematic. I don't want
a shooting pain to hit me at any point where I need to be
steady.

So far, with the help of the Advil, I have managed.

Will pause now. I expect to continue later tonight or tomorrow. In the next section, I thought I would describe a typical Sunday morning now that Kyle's goals have been reached.

Late Tuesday afternoon, classical music from the Interlochen radio station filling the room.

On the way back from town this afternoon after grocery shopping, my car sound system was playing music from my old MP3 player. More specifically, it was playing albums in alphabetical order. The browse album function does not respond when the car is moving, so I let it do what it wanted to do when the album I had chosen a couple of days ago ended. That album was Ray Charles's *Genius Loves Company*. So, the alphabetically minded system moved on to Coltrane's *Giant Steps*, which accompanied me back and forth to town. It finished when I was almost in sight of home and transitioned to Paul Simon's *Graceland* as I drove into my driveway.

During my drives back and forth to town I was struck by Coltrane's music in my ears, its mournful, sometimes seemingly nervous complexity, and outside my car the hills, orchards, and blue waters of the bay flashing by in a restful panorama.

A striking contrast. That somehow suggests how Carol and I now live betwixt and between our then and our now, not quite finding our footing, just as the probing, unsettled and unsettling music coming out of Coltrane's horn is at odds with a landscape that speaks of eons of continuity.

Carol is asleep in her bed, the dog dozing on the floor. A combination of Advil and the activity of a shopping day seems for the while to have eased my back discomfit.

And so I'll do a bit of writing, picking up where I left off. Which was to describe a typical Sunday morning in my world as created by Kyle and his wonderful chair.

Sunday mornings begin the same as the other six days. I usually rouse somewhere between six and eight. I rouse. I do not get up. I am not a naturally early riser. But the combination of sunlight working through the blinds, and my awareness of Carol sleeping in her bed a few feet away begins my waking. Sometimes Carol vocalizes in some fashion. When she finds her left hand through the rails on her bed, she becomes afraid, perhaps because she cannot easily guide the hand back out. That causes a cry of distress. Other times, she laughs at some thought. Most often, though, what I hear is her labored, open-mouthed breathing.

Which in its forceful expression of life is a welcome sound.

Once up, I greet her and assess how much work I will have to do to ready her for the day, and then do whatever is necessary.

On the other six days, I would then effect Carol's transfer to the chair, and head into the kitchen for breakfast.

That is the first tangible indicator that we are in Kyle's world. Previously, I would just go myself into the kitchen to prepare Carol's breakfast and then bring it back to her and serve it to her while she remained in the bed.

But we're talking about Sunday.

On Sundays, I throw some clothes on, leave Carol in her bed, get in the car and drive the four and a half miles to the market where I buy her blueberry muffin, and, if I am lucky, the *Times* will have arrived, and I will pick that up as well. If not, I resign myself to reading the paper online, and head back home. All of that takes about fifteen minutes, a brief enough time to leave Carol in the care of the dog.

Back home, I now move Carol into the chair and then wheel her to the kitchen table. Her breakfast is the same as other days—melon or banana, breakfast sausage, juice—but the muffin is in place of the usual toast with blueberry jam.

And because it is Sunday, after serving breakfast to Carol, and then feeding the dog, and letting her out for her morning constitutional, I toast a frozen bagel, which I had left out to defrost before my trip to the store.

For me, a bagel on Sunday morning is a requirement. Even a frozen bagel. Fortunately, the market stocks a product that claims to have been baked in New Jersey and is actually an almost acceptable substitute for the freshly baked ones I grew up on.

The radio is tuned to *Sunday Morning Baroque* while we all eat. When we're done, I wheel Carol back to the living room, and turn on the old boom box sitting on the piano away from the interference of the cordless phone so the music can continue into the room with us. I read the *Times* if I have it, or leaf through the Sunday edition of the local paper if I don't. I'll get to the online version of the *Times* a little later. When Carol settles back to sleep in her chair, I wheel her to the bed and transfer her back into it.

And thus is our Sunday morning.

In Kyle's world.

Which is different in that Carol now eats breakfast in the kitchen, as do I. We are functioning in a way that resembles our pre-dementia life. The chair makes this imitation possible.

It is one more stay against the inevitable conquest of the disease.

And I am very happy for it. Carol, too, seems more alert and more of the present moment.

The dog has not offered her opinion. Wherever we eat she waits for something to fall to her on the floor.

Sometimes I am envious of a life governed by such simplicity.

Dark Thoughts

Saturday afternoon, humid and cloudy, rain possible, even another thunderstorm as we experienced last night. Carol asleep in bed after the morning in her chair.

I have not been out to check my garden in a few days. Last I looked the beans had not come up yet. Each year I usually have to plant them two or three times before they arise. I don't know why. Maybe the ground has to reach a certain temperature. I think the garden is going to have to accept my relative indifference to it this season.

Or not.

On Thursday when I returned from working for an hour or so at the community library, I found the aide checking out the new book I had started reading and had left, as I always do, on the coffee table.

The book is a new biography by Erica Wagner of Washington Roebling, who took over the supervision of the construction of the Brooklyn Bridge after his father, John Roebling, the designer of that now world famous structure, died slowly, and painfully, from tetanus after refusing appropriate medical treatment for an accident that smashed his foot.

Clearly, I am somewhat familiar with that part of the younger Roebling's life, having read David McCullough's account of the bridge's construction. I am always interested in things related to my hometown of Brooklyn, and that bridge is central to Brooklyn's identity. At the time of its construction it was a groundbreaking engineering miracle, and it is still a compellingly beautiful structure.

This wandering introduction does intend to lead somewhere.

So, here it is.

Naturally, as the retired English professor and present-day writer that I am, I was perfectly happy to see the aide exploring the book. I know she is taking college classes in the nursing program in the community college in town. Wanting to indicate my approval of her looking at my new book, I started talking to her about the bridge. Not surprisingly, given her aspirations to become a nurse, she was perhaps most interested in the senior Roebling's death from tetanus.

Undeterred, I showed her how the bridge appears in the print of the Brooklyn Heights Promenade hanging over the fireplace. She finally got the opportunity to break into my Brooklyn chatter to say, yes, she had seen the bridge herself years ago on a trip to New York.

We are approaching the point.

Which I can articulate no better than to say in the words of the old cliché, what goes around comes around.

Looking at that print, then Carol in her bed not far from it, stirs my memory of that time, previously referenced, when she was living in Brooklyn and when I came in to spend some time with her, we would often dine in a café on Montague Street, and after eating, we would walk to the Promenade and sit on a bench very much like the one in the print and look out at New York Harbor, and of course at the bridge, visible on the lower right, spanning it.

But I do not mean to dwell on either that or Brooklyn, although doing so is perfectly natural for me, and no doubt tedious to anyone else.

Rather, I am thinking of other patterns of repetition. This morning when I wheeled Carol into the kitchen, I was struck by the thought that my father, at about my age, wheeled my mother around because of her arthritic knees. She was about ten years younger than he, as I am ten years older than Carol.

My sister, too, was wheelchair bound, as a result of crippling back difficulties. My brother-in-law pushed her around in her chair.

One way of looking at these circumstances is to attribute them to coincidence and leave the matter comfortably there.

But the way certain associations from the past continue to

reassert themselves into the present offers the possibility of another explanation.

Karma?

But that would suggest some kind of cause/effect patterning.

My mother and sister died young. And Carol is in the grip of this hideous disease.

So, I don't want to go there.

Let's just say thoughts to occupy a rainy afternoon.

And leave it at that.

Monday afternoon. Rain continues. I shut off the irrigation system. Carol noisily but deeply asleep. A good eating day so far, full breakfast, and, unusually, a good lunch of a yogurt, protein bar, and glass of juice. Ryan will likely be here later, and I guess we'll go with pizza. I had thought about grilling some burgers, but that will have to wait for better weather.

Yesterday was Father's Day. I always take a low-key approach to holidays, so I was not particularly disappointed that Carol could not share this day with me. On the other hand, I was happy to speak with my three daughters, Danielle in Brooklyn Park, (I take note of the name) Minnesota, and Tracy and Kerri from Kerri's house in Woodbury, Long Island where she and her sister's family gathered for a barbecue. That provided an opportunity to receive greetings from grandkids as well.

Those conversations took place in the evening at a time when the long, solitary weekend was drawing to its close, so they were especially welcome.

But, as pleasant and welcome as they were, they also stirred up thoughts of my future. Increasingly, I find it difficult to see where I will spend my remaining years. Carol's longevity might take that decision out of my hands, for she will be here, either with me in our house, as now, or in a facility. In either case, I, too, will be here.

So, my thoughts this gray afternoon as to my future contemplate the possibility of Carol predeceasing me.

I don't dwell on such thoughts. They just seem apt in part by yesterday's contact with my daughters, and in part perhaps because of the absence these past few days of the sun.

I do not know, nor does Danielle, where she will wind up. I don't think she feels the pull to come back here. It would be nice if things worked out whereby she could live close to me, but that seems unlikely.

My New York families are rooted there.

These ideas are beginning to whirl around in my head, so I will pause here to let them settle down.

Thursday evening. I am keeping one eye on the NBA draft to see whom the Knicks will pick. I don't follow college basketball, so I have no knowledge, and therefore no preferences. But I have been following the Knicks since I listened to games on the radio when they had players named Ray Felix, Sweetwater Clifton, and Ernie Vandeweghe, and I talked with my father about the chances of the team reaching a hundred points. That was a long, long time ago.

An eventful day, including a visit from the nurse practitioner who found Carol to be in good physical condition. She congratulated me on the job I was doing and talked about whether or when I should consider a respite break of a week or two. She understood my lack of enthusiasm for that idea now, unless I used it to take a trip, perhaps to New York, or Minnesota to visit daughters. That does appeal to me more than banging around this empty house and visiting Carol in a facility.

Highlight of the day, though, was lunch with Archie, an elementary and high school classmate back in Brooklyn, now living downstate but up here for a few days. He raised the question of whether I would return to New York, something he has thought about.

Today is also Danielle's birthday, and talking to her, along with Archie's question, brings me back to where I left off thinking and writing a few days ago.

Which involves musing about my future.

My immediate future is clear. I continue as I am now, perhaps with the addition of a respite trip. In that regard, it seems to me that Carol has plateaued. I don't see much deterioration in her condition. I recognize living so intensely in this situation makes it difficult to notice change, but still I don't think there has been much. In consultation with the nurse practitioner today, we fine-tuned her meds, but nothing very dramatic. We removed the anastrozole, the hormone suppressor that was part of her post breast cancer regimen. Doing so was a hardheaded concession to a possible recurrence of cancer in light of her being in the grips of her present disease. Unstated was the thought that should that happen it might just be better to let that disease take its course. We made a couple of other minor adjustments but nothing indicative of a change in her condition that had to be addressed.

However, beyond that clear present is the much cloudier future.

I am setting up a trust to deal with Carol's needs should I predecease her.

That, too, is clear and necessary.

But what about the reverse. Carol predeceases me. I am ten years older, but in fairly good condition while her disease will likely shorten her life, by an indeterminate, and at this point, impossible to predict degree.

Some time ago, I thought, briefly, about her funeral arrangements. I first did so when one or two people suggested to me that I consider hospice for her. That suggestion, though I am sure it was offered with the best of intentions, has proved to be seriously premature. My thinking about her funeral started and ended with the idea that I would arrange something befitting this place and her family background, which is fundamentally different than mine.

I am content to leave it at that.

And I'll just peek into the room in which resides the vexing question of the arrangements for my own demise, in particular, where I want to be buried or at least memorialized for I am sure I want to be cremated. Spending thousands of dollars on a coffin seems ludicrous to me. In one sense, this ultimate decision is, of course, a matter of supreme indifference to me. But in another way, one that I need to deal with, I should think about those I will be leaving behind. Where should my remains and/or memorial be?

Here where Carol will be, and where we have two graves reserved for us, or Long Island where my family is?

Impossible to know where Danielle will be, and how would she feel if her mother and father were separated in death?

I confess I cannot come to a decision at this time.

So, I will, again, shut that door.

Past, Present, and Future

Sunday night, late. Just going to jot down a few words, so I'll have a place to start, perhaps tomorrow.

On the front page of today's *Times* book review section were the openings of two retrospective looks at *To Kill A Mockingbird*.
I never read it. Saw the movie but did not read the book.
It was, however, Carol's favorite book.

That's the start. Let's see where it goes.

Tuesday evening. Carol in bed and will soon be asleep. Will try to pick up the thread.

When it became clear that Carol would no longer be able to read because her eyes would not stay focused on one line of type, I decided to see if she would listen to an audiobook. The first one I took out of the library was *Mockingbird*, to which she listened attentively, often smiling at something Scout, the young girl narrator of the story, said. I am fairly certain that her love for the book had everything to do with Scout. Maybe she saw something of herself in that character. Perhaps, to go a step further, she also responded to Scout's attachment to Atticus as an idealized version of her relationship with her own father.

I don't think she paid as much attention to the novel's depiction of racism. She was a little conflicted on that issue. Of course, she deplored racism, but she also loved her southern mother who proudly had the stars and bars on the front license plate holder of her car. Her mother does not have a mean bone in her body, but she did grow up in Virginia and most likely just accepted without malice the South's treatment of people of color.

After the success of her listening to the audiobook, I

brought home *Go Set A Watchman*, the then recently published novel, rejected when offered to publishers, but that when rewritten became *Mockingbird*. Carol did not listen as attentively to that book. I don't think we got all the way through it. I tried other audiobooks by her favorite authors, such as Louise Erdrich, but they did not capture her attention.

Mockingbird was special, in part for the reasons already mentioned, and perhaps also because hearing it triggered her memories of having read it.

It was, and perhaps still is, quintessentially her book.

It is not mine. Both reviews in this past week's *Times*, while recognizing the book's status and accomplishment, also take a somewhat less than positive view of how it deals with the racial issue. I don't intend to go into that argument other than to say it does not explain my relative indifference to the book.

For a variety of reasons, I was not drawn to it. Although when it came out in 1960 it soon became almost universally installed on high school reading lists, at that time I was a struggling pre-engineering student at Brooklyn College. I don't recall paying much attention to it then. Within a year I realized that I was swimming upstream in the engineering curriculum and switched to English as my major. I focused on American literature, but Harper Lee's book did not appear on any assigned college or graduate reading lists.

I can't recall when I saw the movie, whether in a theater or on television. I enjoyed the movie, liked the cardboard virtue of Atticus and the sass of Scout, but not in any intense way. I just wasn't moved to pick up the book, as sometimes I did, and do, after first viewing a film based on a novel.

When I saw the reviews in the *Times*, my first thought, quickly abandoned, was I've got to show these to Carol.

A futile idea of course.

Monday night. I have not written much the past few days

for several reasons, beginning with a weird allergic attack that caused my skin to break out in blisters that required steroids to quiet it down. At about the same time I was preparing for the arrival of Tracy and her family Saturday night, getting them settled in on Sunday, and then dealing with a thunder and lightning storm Sunday night that knocked out our power for about six hours.

A week later on Monday afternoon, settling into the usual routine after a week's visit from Tracy and family that filled the house with energy, warmth, and good feelings. Grandkids, not surprisingly, are growing, their personalities emerging and becoming clearer. Watched two or three episodes of The Staircase *with Tracy and found we did not see the murder case in that documentary the same way. Talked politics with Fred, and finally, enjoyed the antics of Dylan, their family beagle who formed a relationship with our Daisy, urging the old Golden to play.*

Although my writing routine was predictably and happily interrupted during my family's visit, I see that I did find the time to leave myself a note about an email from the Shaw Festival. Will sew that thought into the Mockingbird *thread.*

At about the same time as the reviews of *Mockingbird* appeared, a notice about the upcoming Shaw Festival, which we attended some years ago, arrived in my inbox. Both of these threads, *Mockingbird* and the festival, share a common thrust: they are intrusions from the past, insistent reminders of what has been lost. Carol's favorite book, on the one hand, and on the other a vacation trip made all that more special by the fortuitous circumstance of finding that our very good friends, Lowell and Sheila, on the grounds of whose house we were married, were also going to the festival at Niagara-on-the-Lake the same time we were.

As is so often now the case, these memories are bittersweet, with the first part of that oxymoronic word more prominent. I could not, in any meaningful way, talk to Carol about either the book or the festival.

There really is nothing more to be said on that point, and I don't want to start wading into the waters of self-pity, so I will move on.

On the Friday before Tracy and family arrived, a draft copy of the trust I am setting up came in the mail. This morning I emailed my attorney with a few questions I would like answered.

I will pause here, take a figurative breath, and dive into this intensely difficult subject when next I sit down to write.

Mockingbird insists on getting my attention. Its author appears as a clue in today's Times's *crossword puzzle. I have inserted Harper Lee's name in the puzzle and will move on, which in this case means working the puzzle.*

Wednesday, early afternoon, an unusual writing time, but Carol is asleep, and since breakfast was late, lunch won't be for a while. Yesterday was a full day, shopping, Ryan for supper, and so I wasn't up for sitting down with my laptop late as I had planned. Try to make up some ground today.

I am setting up the trust for the obvious reason that I want to be sure that Carol will be well provided for should I predecease her. Of course, being ten years older, I thought that would be the case, and having designated my beneficiaries, starting with her, the only vexing question was where I was to be buried, in Michigan or New York. That question remains, but Carol's no long being competent and requiring care opens up a whole range of unanticipated questions for which I was, and am, unprepared to answer, but which, nonetheless, insist on being presented to me.

I have discovered, not surprisingly, that this is a particularly lonely activity. My attorney and financial advisor can tell me *how* to do what I want, but neither they, nor anybody else, can help me decide *what* I want.

So, I begin with the need for Carol's care, and thus the trust. A trust must have a *settler*, the entity—in this case me—that establishes the trust, and then a *trustee*—again in this case, me during my lifetime—who manages the trust. As such I determine the assets that go into the trust. Apparently, I will also create a pour-over will to deal with assets that are not in the trust when I die. In my case, I imagine these will be mostly personal items.

That's about as much as I now understand, pending answers to questions, and/or confirmations of what I think I understand from my attorney.

None of the above is particularly troubling to deal with, even a bit interesting, as the law has always fascinated me, in part because as a word person I appreciate the law's attempt to provide precise relationships between language and the world. I had a glimpse into that attempt when Carol worked her way to her JD.

Seeing Carol's JD on the wall is a painful reminder of the was, just like the copies on her bookshelves of the journals containing her stories.

But that is not what I am talking about now. Perhaps I am letting myself be distracted.

So, to refocus, the technicalities, the legalisms, of my trust appeal to me on an intellectual level.

However, the decisions those technicalities involve are the ones that are emotionally fraught, and ones I need to deal with by myself.

They include successor trustees, who will be responsible for Carol's care when I am gone, and the ultimate distribution of assets that will remain after that care is no longer necessary.

Those questions are complicated by the fact of there being children from two marriages, and an anticipated inheritance coming to Carol from her family.

I have always posited fairness and equal treatment as the cornerstones of my parenting responsibilities. I still do.

The application of that doctrine in the present and future is the challenge.

And I must handle it alone.

Pulling Back the Curtain

Saturday late afternoon on a warm and muggy day in mid-July. The weather has been hotter than I recall it being during the fifteen previous summers we've lived here. Rocco is across the road spraying loosener on his trees preparing them to be harvested by shaking.

Carol, the first woman shaker driver, on the Peninsula, is sleeping now, and I have some time before preparing supper.

Music playing from Interlochen, and I find that I am wearing an ancient T-shirt, on the front of which is the image of a grand piano and some bars of music, and on the back the word "Dad." Clearly, the shirt was a gift from one of my daughters, but I no longer can recall which. I had forgotten I had the shirt until this morning when I found it on the bottom of the pile of possibilities in my drawer. It feels a little tight, so perhaps I was thinner when I received it. Or it was not correctly sized by the buyer. Or it shrank. None of which helps identify the giver. But what is clear, the choice of the images reinforces the centrality of music in my life.

Which leads to a thought I've been playing with for the past few weeks. Some time ago, Kyle said something to the effect that he would love to know what was going on in Carol's mind. Of course, on a basic level, none of us ever fully knows the workings of another person's mind. We guess based on all kinds of factors, and in the best relationships we probably come pretty close to getting what our mate is thinking. In those relationships, we soon enough find out if we were right or wrong.

But Carol's dementia provides a whole different, much more impenetrable barrier, made even more so by her loss, for the most part, of the ability to articulate her words. She still can provide one-word responses, mostly of the yes or no variety, and even the occasional full sentence, as one of the aides reported her saying "I like watermelon," when being offered that as part of her lunch.

To further complicate matters, as Kyle also explored, it is not possible to know what exactly she sees. I have known for quite some time that the communication between her eyes and her brain has been compromised by the disease. That is why she can no longer read. And why when on the occasions I have her with me in the television room, she listens, but does not look at the screen.

Yet, she still does seem to be looking at things, such as at my face when I lean over her. Waving a hand, as Kyle once did, in front of her eyes produces a defensive closing of them. So, I can conclude that the images sent to her brain by her eyes do stimulate a response, but the nature of that response is not at all clear.

Perhaps some sort of sophisticated neurological testing could provide an answer.

Or maybe not.

These thoughts are just the beginning of an exploration of what is going on in Carol's mind.

Moving away from the visual to the auditory reveals a clear difference. She does process auditory cues, be they in the form of words or music. In terms of the former, she does respond not only to remarks or questions aimed directly at her, but also to what she might hear from others' conversation or even the words floating out into the room from the television or radio. I am also sure, by observing her facial expressions and occasional movements of her hands, that she responds to music.

And still I am only scratching the surface of the question. Deeper questions remain. Kyle has talked about, for example, her loss of the executive function of her brain, so that more primitive impulses are no longer constrained and emerge to create their own responses. Her fear of falling might arise from that situation. The loss of memory in dementia is clearly another obvious factor. But what replaces those lost memories? Is each day a new experience, and if not, to what extent is it not?

In raising these questions, we are trying to get inside the dementia.

Which, no doubt, is impossible.

I've taken this as far as I can for now. Perhaps I'll dig further.

Or perhaps not. It is a scary place to be.

Monday night. Carol snoring, dog sleeping. Just watched Netflix documentary Evil Genius about a most bizarre murder/bank heist case involving a pizza delivery man with a pipe bomb fastened around his neck as the unwilling bank robber in one plot line, and a murdered man found in a freezer on another. Somehow the two plots will meet, and all will be revealed. Too weird to be instructive of anything but distractedly interesting.

And a little distraction is a good thing. I take it where I can find it.

As I often do, I just want to start what follows, enough so I will be able to let it percolate a little bit more, and then wade into it.

In my attempts to understand Carol's dementia, to imagine what it must be like from inside her head, I have been thinking the word "fog" describes her mental state.

But it occurs to me that might be wrong, and therefore misleading.

A fog suggests an environment lacking clarity, where things cannot be seen easily, or perceived at all, if the fog is thick enough. And because Carol often does seem somehow to lack understanding of where she is, the word at first glance seems apt.

But I have been observing indicators that suggest otherwise. It's not so much an inability to perceive her present circumstances, but rather that her mind is elsewhere. And that elsewhere might be perfectly clear to her.

For example, sometimes when I am offering food to her, she seems unaware that eating is her immediate activity. I then say her name with some emphasis, and she starts as though she is being brought back to the present moment and takes a bite of the piece of toast I have been holding in front of her mouth.

A start. Wading into deep waters. Don't want to drown.

Wednesday afternoon. A very noisy and somewhat busy day. Outside, a constant stream of farming-related vehicles, forklifts, tractors, and various-sized trucks, all part of the ongoing cherry harvest. In addition there are the tourist vehicles in an unending procession north to the lighthouse, and south back to town, as well as the mostly quiet packs of cyclists, whose riders' voices sometimes carry into the house as they zip by—all of it almost making me impatient for the quiet of winter when the only vehicles are the snowplows roaring by knocking down the occasional mailbox

Almost.

The phone, too, has been ringing all day, telemarketers and political robocalls as we approach primary day. Among these I finally received one of those scam calls I've read about, an automated voice in the most somber tones instructing me that it is from the IRS, which has issued an arrest warrant for me, and I'd better call the specified number. Immediately. Or be ready to be fitted for an orange perp suit. I don't know whether I should be amused that I have reached the age where I am deemed a target for such a transparent fraud or insulted that it is thought I would fall for it. In that vein, I also received a call from somebody who claimed to have heard I was interested in getting my book published and offered me some help in doing that. Having published fourteen books, I felt like calling this one back and suggesting he update his list.

Friday afternoon, and I am in the community library again for the first time in weeks. None of my lunch companions were available, so after dining alone, and with more time available, I came here to do a bit of writing. I'll see if I can move on into my speculations about what it might be like being in Carol's head.

The library is unusually active, perhaps because of the book sale in an adjoining area. There are a few patrons checking the shelves. A couple of voices in animated conversation float back here from the front desk. To my left, a businessman asks if it is okay with me if he makes a quick phone call. I assure him that he can.

I note that there may be a tactile component to Carol's connection to the here and now.

For example, she seems to enjoy holding hands. She always did. Now, when I take her hand, she squeezes mine as she used to do and does not let it go easily. If I offer her my other hand, she takes it and holds both with some pressure.

I do this most usually when she is lying flat on her back in bed, so I cannot think she holds on to my hands with such intensity because she is afraid of falling. When I release my hands from her grip, she remains comfortably lying there as she was before.

So, what is going on during this simple activity?

More noise coming from the front of the library. It is almost getting to be distracting, even for one such as myself so used to blocking out background noise. A toddler's complaining voice rises above the din. In spite of the distraction, I am happy to see so much activity in the library.

Of course, I can only guess. Perhaps the feel of my hands in hers gives her some sort of comfort or security. I do not think, although I would like to, that she knows the hands holding hers are mine, that they belong to the Steve she seems sometimes to still associate with me, or her memory of me.

In a similar fashion, when I have her sitting on the edge of the bed preparatory to helping her stand so that I can guide her the couple of feet to her chair, she first grabs my shirt or pants. That action clearly arises out of fear of falling.

But then when I put my arms around her in a kind of an embrace so that I will be able to get her onto her feet, she rests her head on my chest. She is calm at that point, perfectly comfortable. It is hard to reject the idea that she knows she is in my arms as she had been so often for so many years.

I talk to her throughout this process.

But she does not vocalize anything with the exception of an objection to being turned around on the bed as I get ready to help her sit up.

So, I am left guessing.

I conclude a couple of things, recognizing that all of this is the purest speculation, not a little colored by what I would like to think is going on.

First, although there might be a little element of fear of falling throughout, I do not think it is significant.

Second, she seems to enjoy the physical intimacy, particularly of my arms around her.

Third, and most important, throughout this process, she seems to be in the moment.

Does she know who is helping her?

I can't answer that.

Does she appear to be confused? In a fog?

No.

When I ease her into her chair, and I am no longer touching her, then, she looks a little confused, as though trying to orient herself to where she is.

I can add one other factor.

The auditory one.

As I mentioned, I talk to her during this process. I first tell her we are about to have breakfast. And I indicate the menu. It always includes breakfast sausage, juice, toast with blueberry jam, and then some kind of fruit: banana, melon, strawberries, or pineapple chunks.

Sometimes I get a response, a little smile, or nod, or even a word or two. Often, not. It seems to me at that point, she is not fully engaged in the present moment.

Meaning in her head, she had been somewhere else.

Not in a fog.

Just somewhere else that made more immediate sense than my prattling about the breakfast menu.

Respite time almost up and I have gone about as far as I can on this speculative subject for now. My companion, the businessman, is still hunched over his laptop. I'll pack up and head home.

Monday night. It's raining again, as it has been doing off and on the past few days. At least the oppressive heat is gone for now.

Yesterday, in spite of my earlier decision to give up on keeping the piano tuned, I had Brant come out again to fix the E above middle C key. He did that and more, devising a way to lubricate the action so the keys wouldn't stick, all the while talking to himself, or his tools, or perhaps the piano. He loves to talk, about all kinds of things, such as his discovery of a way to plant potatoes on top of the soil.

Given how starved for conversation I usually am on week-ends, the dog being particularly useless in this regard, I was happy to hear what he said on that and various other topics including environmental poisons of which we are unaware.

After he leaves, I sit down at the keyboard and reintroduce myself to Gertrude and her waltz by pecking out the notes in the first few bars. She does not seem to mind, nor does she appear to be happy to see me back.

Not a lot of energy tonight, so I will just try to get back into my thoughts concerning what is happening in Carol's head.

At supper last night, without planning to do so, I held Carol's hand with my right hand while with my left I held the fork of food in front of her mouth. I can't say why I did that, never having done it before during meals. I do like to hold her hand because she returns the pressure and sometimes seems reluctant to let my hand go. On other occasions, she will put her other hand on mine as well so mine is enclosed between hers.

I do not know what to make of this. Perhaps her actions are no more than neurological responses having nothing to do with any thought process or emotion. Or maybe they represent her happiness with the flesh-to-flesh contact. In that respect, I frequently hold her hand(s) as she is going to sleep, perhaps fidgeting as she sometimes does, and it seems to me doing that calms her down, eases her into a sleep mode as she closes her eyes.

Of course, I can be making too much of some or all of this.

But I am not so sure.

Perhaps these moments of physical intimacy stir pleasant memories.

When I took her hand at supper, I think it was because, as often is the case, her hands were waving about. I believe at those times she simply cannot control them. Maybe I just took her hand to stop it from moving about in the vicinity of the fork with food on it.

In any case, she squeezed my hand and the involuntary motions stopped.

Absent a better explanation, I will permit myself to believe there is some intent on her part to feel her flesh against mine.

Did You Miss Me?

Wednesday late after an uneventful day.

A brief but provocative conversation this morning.

After serving Carol her breakfast and feeding the dog hers, I started fixing mine. I realized that in my grocery shopping yesterday, I had forgotten to get milk, this even though I have downloaded a very serviceable shopping list app. I discovered, however, the list is useless if you don't enter an item on it. So, although I knew I needed milk, I didn't see it on the list on my phone and did not buy it.

All of which is preface to my deciding that because I really wanted milk for my cereal, I would hop in my car and drive to the market. I can usually make it to the market and back in about fifteen to twenty minutes and feel reasonably comfortable in leaving Carol alone in the house with the dog for that length of time.

Carol was sitting in her chair in the living room with classical music from the Interlochen station playing. "I'm going to the store," I said, "and will be back in a few minutes."

She didn't respond, which is not unusual. In those situations, I do not know whether she has processed what I have said. Perhaps she was so into the music, or even somewhere else in her mind, that my words did not register.

No matter. She was securely belted into the chair. Nothing bad was going to happen in those fifteen or twenty minutes, so off I went.

Even though I had to cross a double yellow line to get by a one-man cherry shaker doing about five miles per hour, I was back within those fifteen minutes. I walked into the living room, leaned over Carol, kissed her forehead, and said, "I'm back."

At first, she did not respond.

"Did you miss me?" I said.

And here's the point of my describing this incident.

"Yes," she said. "I did."

Let's take a closer look at that response.

The first word, the affirmation, does not indicate much. She could have recognized that she was being asked a yes/no question, and so picked one of the two appropriate responses.

But her unprompted continuation offers a more provocative possibility. It declares that she knew what I was asking and wanted to be sure she told me that.

Now, I don't want to push this analysis too far. My question was not serious, having been gone for so short a time. My voice might have indicated that I was teasing her.

But I will go this far in the context of my attempts to imagine her brain's activity to suggest that she moves back and forth between a connect and disconnect with the here and now.

As do we all. Only for those of us not afflicted with dementia we are much more in tune with the here and now, even when our minds, or part of our minds, are somewhere else.

I guess my question for Carol is where her mind is when it is so fully disconnected from the here and now. It is somewhere.

But where is that somewhere?

Sunday night after a quiet weekend interrupted by virtually no human contact. I believe I say that almost every time I sit down to work after a weekend. However, the repetition doesn't make that observation any the less true.

And as usual, the only face-to-face interaction this weekend occurred on my Sunday morning trip to the store. I arrived a little later than usual, partly by design, and was rewarded by finding out that the Times *had just arrived. I miss reading from the physical paper rather than following links on my computer screen. I find I dig deeper when I have all those sections sitting in my lap.*

While in the store I checked, as I do only very occasionally, to see the status of the copies of my books being offered for sale, hoping to attract the attention of the summer visitors as the locals have already had ample opportunity to purchase them. I noticed that the books were hidden behind a cart laden with ears of corn. There is a metaphor lurking in this situation, but I haven't discovered it. Anyway, I alerted the regular clerk who moved the cart so that my titles were again visible.

I have been exploring what I imagine to be the interior of Carol's brain. I have concluded that it is an active place, a workshop of ideas, and/or memories that prompt responses such as a sudden, inexplicable burst of laughter as if she had told herself a joke or just remembered something amusing. At other times, she seems to be forming words, but they are not clearly enough articulated for me to understand them.

What I want to add to this exploration is recognition of her marvelous imagination that provided her the material for her stories. I think it likely that her imagination continues to generate ideas even in her present impaired state. Why would it not? Why would it shut down?

Quite often her facial expression certainly looks as though she is deep in thought. True, I sometimes think she is focused on the music that is coming from the radio. But that is not an adequate explanation for that expression, which also does occur absent any music reaching her ears.

Something very intense and clear is going on behind that expression. I will never know what that something is, can't even begin to make a guess.

Other than to be reasonably sure that whatever it is, it is the product of that same powerful imagination out of which arose her stories.

And speaking of her stories leads to my very recent decision to see about getting them collected into a book, a project we had, in fact, been working on when she got sick.

Tired. Will pick this up when next I write.

Tuesday night. Usual shopping day. Carol has been eating with more appetite these past few days, and that is a good thing.

Yesterday, I got on the treadmill for the first time in probably almost two years. I have felt a need to get back into regular exercise and hope to be able to continue. Part of the problem is the location of the treadmill in the furnace room in the basement. I like to exercise with music, and I'm concerned about being down there with my music on for forty-five minutes or so. I know I am exaggerating the risk and might even be using it as an excuse not to exercise. A more legitimate impediment to my doing exercise is lack of energy or the need at times to just chill out. I have checked into buying a folding stationary bike to be used in the living room within sight of Carol's bed.

All of this speaks to the problem of finding my footing in these difficult circumstances.

I have begun making inquiries concerning the publication of Carol's stories by sending the beginning of the manuscript containing the first two stories to readers associated with Mission Point Press, which published my recent books. Not surprisingly both these readers wrote back with strong praise for the stories.

As they should.

I will also get in touch with another well-established local writer who has connections with a university press, which would probably provide wider distribution and perhaps more recognition.

Which these stories very much deserve.

Returning to the question of Carol's mental activity now, I wonder if she is still exercising her imagination to write new stories. Sometimes it seems that she is deep in thought about something. If I need her attention on those occasions, I have to call her name a couple of times until she starts, and then responds with a look on her face as though I have pulled her back from the place to which her mind had carried her.

Other times, she suddenly laughs as though having remembered a joke.

Or perhaps has just created one.

Of course, I will never know.

And I deeply regret that there will not be any more of her wonderfully imagined connections to the natural world in which she grew up, the waters of the bay, the farmland carved out of the rolling hills, the flowers and fauna, all of which was so vivid in her stories that the reader is transported into that world.

That world is peopled by the characters she places there, Native Americans, some wise, some comic, or the young farm girl in some of them, no doubt a stand-in for herself looking to move out beyond the borders of that environment.

And always a search for, and insistence on, basic decency, her declared intention being to use her stories to instruct us on how we should live.

So sad that at best, the new incarnations of that fictional world remain locked in a mind that can no longer birth them into the present for us to enjoy and appreciate.

In a strange kind of way that thought, the idea that not only I, but the larger world, suffers a significant loss as a result of her disease, provides a level of comfort to me.

Being robbed of her talent the world can join me in regretting her sliding into the unreachable depths of dementia.

Small comfort indeed.

But I'll take it.

First job as J.D., legal editor at West Publishing. >>>

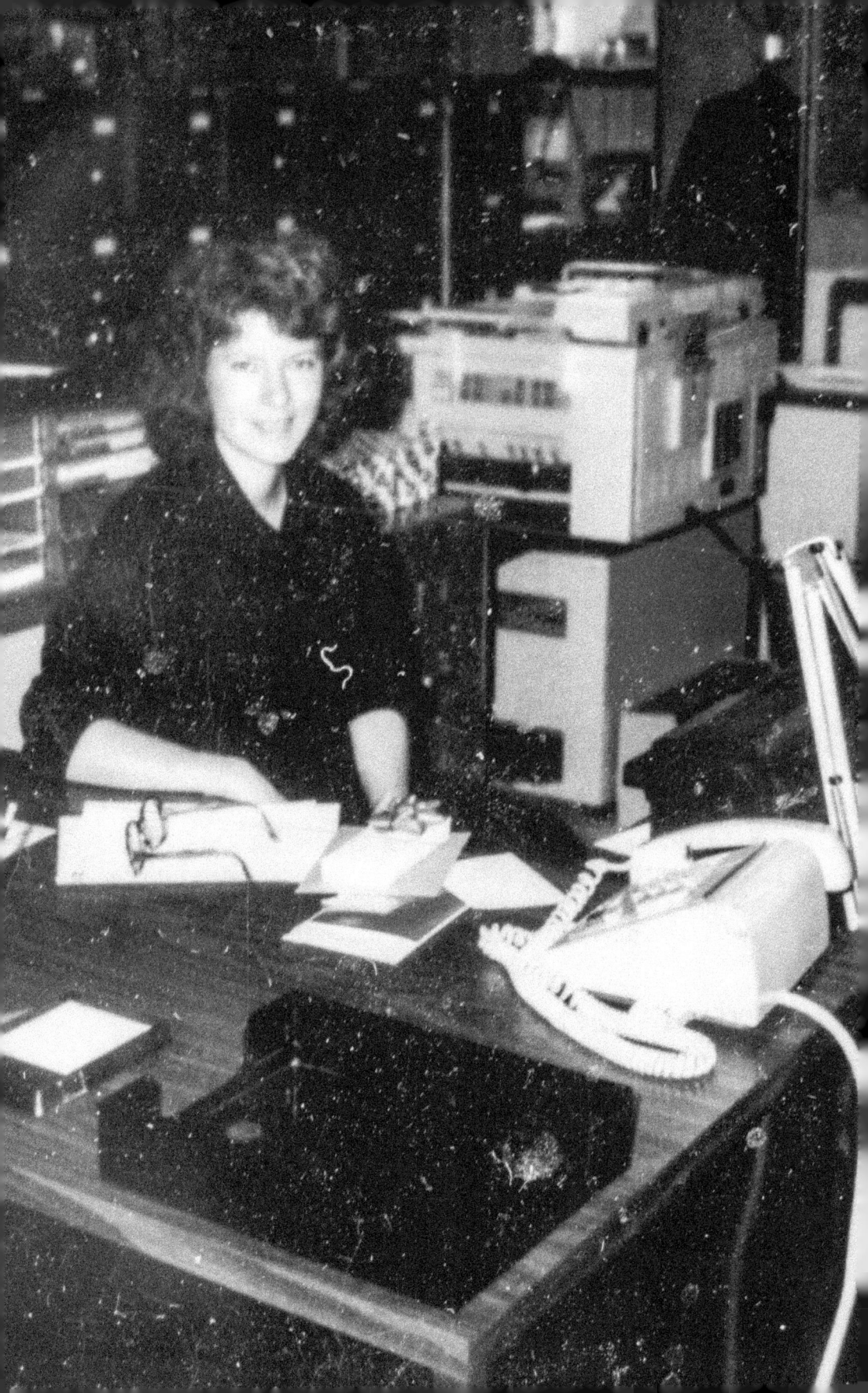

Of Then and Now Redux

Monday night. Carol dozing in her chair after supper. Before long, I will transfer her into her bed for the night. Time enough to start a writing session and see where it might lead.

I've said more than once that weekends, actually the period from Friday afternoon when the week's last relief aide leaves until Tuesday afternoon when the first aide of the week arrives, that four-day stretch is difficult for me, although I doubt Carol is aware. Ryan's Monday night visits for dinner shortened that stretch but he is working six full days in the restaurant during this summer season and comes to mow the lawn and perhaps join us for a meal when he can find the time, usually later in the week.

These last four days have been different. Tomorrow is an election day for primaries for state and local positions, and the phone has not stopped ringing with political robocalls. One such, which my caller ID told me was from Hamtramck, Michigan, by itself caused the phone to ring four times. I did not total the number of such calls, but I am confident that twenty for today alone would be a conservative number.

The calls started slowly on Friday and crescendoed about two hours ago. Not the kind of human interaction I would prefer.

Late Saturday afternoon. Carol and dog sleeping. Just finished the Times *crossword puzzle.*

Through open, screened front door comes the constant sound of traffic going up and down Center Road. Most of the vehicles are clearly those of tourists heading back and forth visiting the lighthouse and Hessler Log Cabin in the park at the north end of the Peninsula. The cars are driving fast along this state road that passes by our house. In the spring, they move more slowly because they are looking for cherry blossoms; in the fall, they also travel at a leisurely pace checking out the colors of the turning leaves. Only in the winter is this road quiet.

Yesterday was our anniversary. It came and went like all other days. Not surprising. Carol and I used to celebrate by going out to eat, usually at an upscale restaurant. We didn't swap presents, nor did we encourage our daughter to congratulate us, which, is, when I think about it, a kind of silly idea anyway. Why would she be congratulating us? For conceiving her?

Maybe I'm being too literal, so I'll leave that point alone.

Because Carol has lost weight, she no longer wears the diamond ring I bought for her years after we married when finances permitted. One day I found it on the couch cushion where she was then sleeping. I figured out a way to have it properly sized by using one of those ties that can be adjusted to a certain circumference. I wrapped one around her ring finger until it fit securely as I would want the ring to do. I thought I would take it and the ring into a jeweler and have the ring downsized.

I gave up on that idea after a while and just put the ring in a safe place. Seeing her finger sans the ring bothered me, but not for long.

I did tell Carol that it was our anniversary. I do not know if she processed that fact. I could not see any obvious reaction.

Some motorcycles just roared by to provide a different external audio. If I were to keep track of the traffic, I would guess this would be one of the busiest days of the year. There is barely an interval of quiet. I need to draw on my ancient city mindset to block it out.

I have been thinking of writing again about what seems to be the central fact of my life now. The thought was prompted, as it usually would be, by the appearance of something, an object, innocent by itself, but emblematic to me.

In this case, the thing appeared when on my way into town I glanced in my rearview mirror and saw hanging from the mirror in the car behind me the kind of handicap placard we used to display, and which I still have in the brown paper bag into which I loaded stuff from the lease car I turned in last December.

There was no point in installing the placard in the new car, so it remains in the bag. Maybe I should just toss it. Somehow, however, that act strikes me as being significant in a way I don't feel like confronting.

Time to think about preparing supper. Will pick this up later.

Sunday night. Watched a repeat of Sherlock *on* PBS. *Forgot how the series had fallen in love with special effects to reveal inner turmoil. Find the technique somewhat distracting and irritating. I prefer my Sherlock straight up.*

Will try to pick up where I left off and see how far my limited energy tonight will carry me.

Seeing that handicap placard in the car behind me and recalling the one we still have now in a paper bag rather than hanging in our car, encapsulates the *then* and *now* mixture ever present in my mind. However, that binary formulation is a little simplistic.

Because the *then*, itself, is composed of various layers. There is the *then* of the time before Carol got sick. Objects reminding me of that *then* are all over the house, in her towel still hanging on the rack next to mine in the upstairs bathroom where I shower, in her glasses, which just the other day I took up to her dresser after they had been lying on the cocktail table in the living room for the past year and more since it became clear that they were no longer needed, in objects small like those and large like the piano she used to play.

I could make a very long list of such objects.

Or in the occurrence in some context of a particular word that resonates because of its association with the Carol of *then*. For example, in a crossword puzzle the answer to one of the clues was "gist." Whenever Carol was trying to puzzle something out, she would say she was after the "gist" of the thing, as though she was seeking the hard kernel of fact or truth hidden somehow from her grasp.

Or a different kind of word association, such as reading in the daily newspaper's column that gathers tidbits from a century ago, the name of Frank Edgecomb. He was Carol's grandmother's first husband. His family built the farmhouse in which Carol grew up. He was not, however, her grandfather. He died in the great influenza epidemic, and Carol's grandmother married the man who became Carol's grandfather.

But Frank was a presence in our house. On the shelf over our bed is a book I bought for Carol about that influenza epidemic, and there is a picture of him on a shelf of the bookcase in the bedroom.

Perhaps more poignant are those things that mark the responses to the increasing debilities of her disease, such as the handicap placard, but also the grab bars in various places in the house, the walker, the shower stool, the shower bench, and the white plastic ruler sitting on the little table between the chairs in the green room, which we thought would enable her to keep her eyes focused on a line of text so that she could continue to read, these and others like them, signposts along the way toward the hospital bed in which she now spends a good portion of her life.

Will try to wrap this up next session by moving into the now into which these objects intrude like guests overstaying their welcome.

Tuesday evening after an eventful day. The morning was ordinary, rising, breakfast, checking in with the world large and small. Once the relief aide arrived, however, things got a little more intense.

I had squeezed in a necessary appointment with my attorney to sign the papers setting up the trust. Of course, that bit of business took longer than I had anticipated as I should have known would be the case based on previous life experiences in which I had spent time conducting legal business.

After leaving the attorney's office, I still had the week's grocery shopping to do. Although I accelerated through that task I could not find, as usually I did, time for lunch out. So I came home, tired and hungry and irritated.

Irritated because the Pandora app in my spiffy new Camry refused to load the program. And worse, as I fiddled with it, it froze in its loading mode and blocked all other audio inputs from working, so I had to drive home in silence.

I had a little rest before the speech therapist arrived to check out Carol's swallowing. More of that below.

After she left and before preparing supper—frozen dinners for both of us—I addressed the Pandora problem in a long telephone conversation with Toyota's tech support only to learn finally, after all strategies failed, that Toyota was aware of, and trying to find a solution to, the problem in the app that is part of its Entune suite. I took small comfort that the problem was now out of my reach. The tech gave me a work-around with which I had to be content.

The visit from the speech therapist was in recognition that difficulty in swallowing is a predictable occurrence in the course of the progression of Carol's disease. On the advice of the nurse practitioner some time ago I began adding a thickener to her liquids to prevent them from eluding the flap that keeps them out of her lungs. Anything that doesn't belong there that gets into the lungs is likely to lead to pneumonia.

But aside from liquids I had noticed that occasionally solid food would get caught in her throat going down, producing a coughing fit and once or twice the forcible expulsion of whatever had been trapped.

My daughter Tracy, who in her practice as a malpractice attorney has become aware of danger signs, had encouraged me to see about having a swallowing test administered as she has seen performed in a hospital setting.

It turns out that kind of test demands a hospital setting. But the therapist did have Carol drink both thickened juice and straight water and observed how her throat managed these. She did not see anything alarming. I also told her what kind of food she ate without problems for the most part, such as chewy protein bars.

All of which leads to turning this line of thought into a positive direction. Belatedly, I had realized that part of Carol's problem was excessive phlegm in the throat. This should have been apparent sooner.

Because I have the same issue, no doubt caused by all the dust and mold in this century-old farmhouse. I find myself blowing my nose throughout the day.

To clear the mucus.

Carol cannot blow her nose.

My theory, confirmed by the therapist, is that the mucus drips down into her throat, or perhaps just gathers there, where it has no place to go and where it becomes a kind of food trap. Supporting this idea, again from my own experience, is that I occasionally have coughing fits from bits of food caught in my throat.

I recalled that my physician some time ago had recommended Claritin for my running nose. I had forgotten that. I found we still had some pills. I began giving them to both of us, once a day.

I blow my nose with less frequency.

And more important, occasional difficulties with trapped food bits have almost disappeared.

That is the beginning of the positive light in our situation.

About done for the night. Will resume with relating a more significant improvement.

Sunshine and Clouds

Monday evening after supper. Carol sleeping in her chair and I will shortly move her into her bed. Just want to get started because I've not been able to find time and ambition over the weekend.

About a week or so ago, when Ryan had joined us for dinner and was still here as I was transferring Carol from the wheelchair to her bed, he witnessed something startling.

I was talking Carol through the steps of the transfer process as I always do. When I reached the part where I say that with my help she will stand up and dance over to the bed, at that point as I started to put my arms around her, but before I began an upward motion, on her own she lifted herself up off the seat of the chair.

And began, albeit unsteadily and uncertainly, to stand.

Let's be clear. Without a doubt she would not have stood all the way up without my usual help.

But she had remembered the routine. She had responded to the verbal prompt.

The next morning, the nurse practitioner was here and witnessed the same thing. She was shocked.

In a good way.

And so, I ask myself, has Carol created a new memory?

If so, how significant is that?

Okay. Got it started.

Tuesday night. Just glanced through a document from my elder attorney which detailed the loose ends that have to be tied up for the trust to be prepared for all contingencies. I confess my earlier interest in the legalism of this business has evaporated and I did not focus as well as I should have. I understand that guarding against unfortunate contingencies is necessary even if my eyes start to glaze as I read about them.

Continuing my exploration of the possibility that Carol has formed a new memory.

Perhaps that is not accurate. I could see what I can find out on this subject by doing the appropriate neurological research.

But I won't.

In the first place, although I know well enough how to do research, I never enjoyed doing it all that much.

Second, I anticipate that the research would not yield a clear consensus since so much about this disease is not yet understood.

So, I prefer to observe and think about what I see.

What is clear is that in starting to stand during our transfer process Carol is responding to a verbal prompt. If I don't say anything, nothing happens.

I have not tried that verbal prompt in other situations. I don't want to muddy those waters. I believe that if there is a new memory, it has a fragile hold in Carol's brain. After those first few successful responses, on other occasions she needed more encouragement from me to begin to stand.

Another complication has also to be factored in. I sense a war going on in Carol's head between her primal fear of falling that still causes her to push back instead of forward and up, and her occasional executive function overcoming that fear. This conflict is most obvious at the beginning of the transfer process when either from the chair or the bed, I move her into a sitting position as a prelude to getting her on her feet. Sometimes this step goes smoothly, but other times she pushes back hard. If I resist that backward movement for a little while and verbally coax her into relaxing, she generally does. Once relaxed, I am guessing that her executive function has asserted itself.

If not that, I don't know what.

The larger point, however, the bigger question, is whether or not her brain even so compromised by this disease has any recuperative possibilities.

Does she, in fact, as I asked at the beginning, retain the ability to make new memories?

Maybe a new memory is not right.

Perhaps her brain is somehow recapturing old information still stored there.

In either case, though, she is doing something she had not been doing for a long time. That in itself is remarkable.

And cause for a little good feeling. I am not foolish enough to expect much more, certainly not any additional improvement.

And as always with this disease, even good news such as this is also a stark reminder of how far down this road, from which there is no real turning back, we have traveled.

In the community library Thursday afternoon. Unusually active, as librarian seems to be introducing a woman and her children to the layout of books on the shelves. Perhaps the family has recently enrolled the kids into the charter school, opening in a couple of weeks, that is replacing the public school in this building.

Pure speculation on my part. But I am a fiction writer, an observer of people, and I do this kind of thinking automatically. And if I choose to write a story about this family, my speculation can be the basis, the skeleton I will have to clothe and provide inner lives to.

I have completed setting up my trust although certain chores remain to finish its implementation, such as designating additional beneficiaries for an insurance policy that lists only me now, and for our joint checking account as well. The trustees will need access to these accounts.

I will take a deep breath before proceeding with those chores.

All of this business turns my mind inevitably toward my own end of life. When my father died some twenty-five or so years ago, I became the last survivor of my nuclear family. An image occurred to me at about that time. I am riding up an escalator with nobody in front of me. I suppose in my imaginings this was my family's private escalator, and ahead of me, having already reached the top and then disappeared, were my mother, sister, and father.

In that order.

They rode up and then they were gone.

For some reason, I do not look back to see who might be coming up behind me. Perhaps I am being self-absorbed.

Or don't want to say good-bye.

But for better or worse, my focus is straight ahead toward that top over which at some point I will go.

And then disappear.

Enough of that kind of dark thoughts this sunny after-noon as my respite period nears its end.

As I start to pack up my laptop, a young boy, one of those who had been introduced to the library, sits down at an adjoining table and looks disapprovingly in my direction, perhaps unhappy with the noise of my opening the case into which I will put my laptop. He has a pile of books on his table. For a few moments, standing in front of him is an older woman, who probably is not related, but just another patron. Still, observing these old and young users of this library provides a kind of antidote to gloomy speculations.

Saturday night. Not really going to start a writing session. Just want to record one incident that fits my exploration of the workings or non-workings of Carol's brain. So here it is.

This afternoon in keeping with my recent commitment to exercise on the treadmill three days a week, one of which would be Saturday, I changed from my sandals into my walking shoes. Carol was in her bed. I leaned over her to tell her that I was going downstairs to the treadmill.

Then I said, "Now, you just stay here." I often say that as a kind of way to thumb our noses at the nasty fates that have made that statement ridiculous. This time I added, "And don't party like you usually do when I'm gone."

Her face opened into a wide smile.

And she laughed.

Not a big belly laugh, but a very discernible laugh.

She was with me in that moment, completely, and as fully as she used to be.

I don't know if I had a lilt to my step, but my upcoming exercise surely seemed less a chore, if not quite a celebration.

Of Memory, Hers and Mine

Tuesday night, late. Not much energy. Violent thunderstorms the past couple of days. One last night knocked our power out not long after I went to sleep at about twelve thirty. I had put the ceiling fan on because the air was so humid. I roused when somehow I realized the fan was not turning. My night's sleep was interrupted for several hours while I retrieved lanterns and a flashlight and tried contacting the power company to tell it that the call I received indicating power was back on did not apply to our house. Power came back on some time later.

Tuesday is my shopping day, so I dragged myself into town and bought groceries. Carol had a bed bath today as she does now every Tuesday and Friday, leaving her tired so I took the opportunity to rest.

More storms are predicted. I have one of the lanterns on the table next to the couch where I can reach it.

Carol's condition seems stable, and in some ways almost a little better. For the most part she eats fairly well and does not resist the necessary handling of her body. She seems to have, as I have observed before, developed new memory capability, in having learned the steps involved in the transfer process, sometimes even anticipating the one when I encourage her to stand up by beginning to rise up off the seat of the wheelchair.

Not always. But often enough to suggest the idea has found a resting place in her brain that can be reached.

She does have occasional difficulty swallowing. But that does not appear to be a neuromuscular issue caused by her disease. Rather, as confirmed by a speech therapist whom I asked to check her out, the difficulty is caused by mucus collecting in Carol's throat because she does not, cannot, blow her nose.

Mucinex has helped relieve her problem.

The well is dry. Will let it fill again and resume, perhaps tomorrow.

Friday afternoon in the community library having popped into town for a follow-up blood test ordered by my doctor. Frankly, I don't recall which of my numbers had shown a slight rise leading to the retest.

Lot of traffic in town, likely because this is the beginning of the last big weekend of the summer leading to Labor Day on Monday.

I ended last time saying that Mucinex has helped relieve the food trap issue for Carol. It has, but not completely. It would have been foolish to think any such problem can be fully eliminated.

On a more positive note, yesterday there was another instance when Carol's mind seemed to have held on to the present moment.

We were finishing breakfast, when she kind of started, as sometimes she does when her brain appears to be refocusing, coming back from wherever her imagination had been taking her.

"Mom," she said, quite distinctly. I was unsure whether she was calling for her mother, as perhaps she had done when she was a child. Her tone did not suggest that.

"Are you thinking of your mother?" I asked.

She nodded.

"She's in Orchard Creek, being taken care of," I said, offering a factually correct response.

"That is good," she said.

She did not seem puzzled by the specificity of the response. Did she remember the facility at Orchard Creek where once when she was still able to travel, we had visited her mother?

Perhaps.

Or maybe she was only indicating she was glad that her mother was being taken care of.

But even that involves her remembering that her mother, indeed, requires care, and can no longer be expected to provide it for her or anybody else.

When I get home, I will mention that at the post office I met an old friend, more hers than mine. I will be curious to see how she responds to his name.

Respite time about over.

She did not respond to her old friend's name, even with a little prodding.

Monday night, late at the end of the three-day Labor Day Weekend during which motorcycles roared up and down Center Road throughout the daylight hours. Maybe there was a biker convention in town. I am sure these vehicles could be made to run more quietly. But the noise is part of the point, isn't it? I recall an incident from years ago when we were living in Centereach on Long Island, New York, in a house that backed on to the power company's easement, an area of sand lanes between scrubby vegetation. Those sand lanes attracted dirt bikers. One day, the noise from those was particularly irritating, and so as one approached, I walked out of our backyard onto the easement and stopped the approaching bike, on which sat a boy of about ten or twelve. "Your bike makes a hell of a lot of noise," I said to him. His expression, which had been apprehensive as he was confronted by an adult male, broke into a broad smile. "Yeah," he replied. I let him think that we were bonding over our mutual appreciation for making a lot of noise.

Carol does not seem to be bothered by the noise even though I am becoming convinced that she is dealing with the world primarily through sound. It is clear to me that she listens intently to the music I have playing, but also the occasional spoken words from the hourly news updates or other commentary. In that regard, I do not believe she retains much information. But if I tell her about something I think she might react to, she sometimes does as when I told her Aretha Franklin, whom we had seen at Interlochen, had died. The fact of Aretha's death registered and produced a facial expression of regret, but the concert we attended did not seem to provoke a memory.

This afternoon, Tracy, back from a trip to Colorado, called. Carol was sleeping, and the music was still playing, so I moved into the green room to talk to my daughter. During the conversation, I heard loud sounds coming from Carol. I couldn't tell if they were cries or laughs. Carrying the phone, I went back into the living room to her bed and heard again what now was clearly boisterous laughter. Tracy heard it as well.

"What's so funny?" I asked Carol. "Did you tell yourself a joke?"

"Yes," she said.

A little later, while I was back in the green room, I heard that laugh again. As did Tracy.

"I'd love to know what that's about," Tracy said.

"So would I," I replied.

And I certainly would.

In fact, although I may be mistaken, I believe Carol has been somewhat more verbal lately, more likely to respond with words, or the occasional sentence.

A pleasant note, to close this writing session.

Wednesday night late. A productive day insofar as I attended to some writing business. I sent off Carol's stories to a university press editor who asked to see the whole manuscript. Turns out she had some preliminary conversation with Carol about the story collection some years ago. And as long as I was in that frame of mind, I sent out two of my stories that still need to find a home.

Then a good supper with Ryan, good because I always enjoy his company, and good because Carol ate well as she had done throughout the day.

Kyle called this afternoon at the suggestion of Clare, the nurse practitioner, who no doubt informed him of Carol's progress in responding to the transfer process by starting to stand. He agreed that this was remarkable and said he would get back to us when he figured out when he could again work with Carol.

I don't know what Kyle might be able to accomplish, but the fact that he thinks it worth pursuing is encouraging.

At dinner with Ryan, Carol again participated in our conversation, laughing at something humorous, and verbally expressing her enjoyment of the Chinese takeout. In this regard, and in a continuation of the seeming improvement in her cognition, she has lately used my name again, which she had not done for some time. It is still not absolutely clear that she associates my name with the physical me, but I am beginning to suspect, perhaps willfully, that she does, at least some of the time.

The past couple of days I have tuned in to the hearings on the Supreme Court nominee. As I sat there, the thought struck me with considerable force that these hearings are something Carol would have loved to watch, combining her law background with her political views.

I suppose these moments when I am reminded of our past time together will continue to pop into my mind, unbidden, and I can choose to welcome them or not.

I hope I have the strength to accept them as a way of being thankful for what we were able to share for so long, to hold onto and cherish those memories and refuse to yield to self-pity at what has been lost.

That is a hard lesson to teach myself.

But I try.

Time

Sunday night. WSHU in my earbuds after watching The Miniaturist *on* Masterpiece. *Apparently, it is a repeat, but I was unaware of that. Set in 17th century Amsterdam, which attracts my interest. Plot premise of some mysterious connection between a model house and the actual house is a stretch, but I will see if it can be made to work.*

The weekend was less isolating than usual, in part because of what I did yesterday, and in part because of what my daughter Tracy did today. Yesterday, I wanted to post something on Instagram for no particular reason other than I now have an account. I noticed that some writers post images of their book covers, so I thought I'd do that. However, I wasn't satisfied with the shots I took because I couldn't get them sized right. So instead, I posted an image of the spines of my eight novels on my bookshelf and shared it with Facebook. That drew some attention and comment.

Today is the first full day of Rosh Hashanah. Carol and I used to invite four good friends and together we would prepare the meal: I would cook the brisket, and Carol would prepare apples and carrots. Our guests would bring something sweet for the new year.

But that was then, and this is now. I am low-keyed about holidays generally, and in spite of those happy memories of sharing the occasion with friends, I was still comfortable letting the Jewish New Year slide by without my notice.

But when I checked my messages this morning, I discovered that I was part of a group message Tracy started through which family members could exchange greetings. I enjoyed participating in the group, which connected me, albeit digitally, to family members in New York; Florida; Manchester, England; California; and even Australia where my cousin Ben is a rabbi.

I'd be dishonest or at least incomplete if I did not mention that today was also a big sports viewing day for me—baseball and football. Won the former, lost the latter.

When I came home Friday, Tonda, the aide, told me that Carol had been very verbal expressing her displeasure as a trainee aide was attempting to give her a bed bath. The immediate point was that this trainee, who otherwise did a good job, might not work out if a bed bath was going to be expected of her were she to be assigned at some point to work here.

More important, however, and Tonda was aware of this, was Carol's being verbal. I have noted that Carol is talking more. She continues, of course, to have articulation problem, but she simply is attempting to speak, or perhaps in her mind she is, in fact, speaking.

In two ways.

She is giving voice to people she is thinking about.

And she is responding more often and clearly to conversational bits that attract her attention.

I have mentioned an example of the first, when without any obvious external stimulation, she said "Mom." When I asked if she were thinking of her mother, she nodded. I responded that she was being taken care of in Orchard Creek, and Carol replied, quite clearly, "That is good."

Then, a day or two ago, while she was sitting in her chair across from where I was in mine working on my laptop, she looked up as if she had remembered something, or a thought had occurred to her, and said "Danielle," our daughter's name. I cannot remember the last time she said that name. I, of course, talk to her about Danielle, usually without much response.

"She is living in Minnesota," I said, "like you did years ago."

She nodded.

On another occasion, in a similar matter, she said "Ward," her younger brother's name.

And this morning while still in bed, she again appeared to be reacting to a thought, and said "Dad."

Finally, in a similar but somewhat different way, recently several times she has addressed me by name, again something she has not done in a while.

I don't know quite what to make of these one-word utterances, other than to say they are new, and they indicate the emergence of some kind of stored memories.

Got this started. Perhaps a good time to let it percolate.

Tuesday night after a long and tiring day including my weekly shopping and a wasted visit to my dermatologist whose office managed to lose my appointment, which I had to reschedule for a couple of weeks down the road.

But the day also offered a couple of bright spots. The first was an email from the editor of Rosebud, *which published one of my stories last winter and to which I sent three more a few days ago. The editor responded to one story in particular commenting on the very last line as not wrapping the story up. I reread the story and concluded he was probably right. I rewrote the ending and sent it off to him. That he took the time to be that specific suggests he might well take the story.*

The second bright spot was a totally unexpected call from Toyota's executive offices to which I had sent an old-fashioned paper letter complaining about my continuing problem with the Pandora app on my Camry's Entune system. I suggested in that letter that my lease fee be reduced by ten dollars a month until Toyota fixed the problem. To my utter surprise someone actually read the letter, took the time to research my previous contacts on the issue, and promised to get back to me by Thursday.

We'll see if this actually goes somewhere.

I've been writing about the apparent improvement in

Carol's ability to pull out shards of long-term memory, such as giving voice to family members, such as her mother, father, and brother, as well as our daughter Danielle, and occasionally calling me by name.

I do not know what, if anything, to make of these brief outpourings.

But I do realize that trying to deal with them, besides guessing at their significance, also puts me in mind of one of the most difficult underlying problems of our situation.

That is how to deal with the persistent push and pull of time, the before of her disease, the now of her condition, and the movement, however haltingly, toward the future.

Simply, I have always had an exaggerated sense of time, even an intense relationship. I hate being late. For anything. In fact, one of the very few sources of disagreement between us was Carol's opposite attitude toward time, in general, and timeliness, in particular. To say we were wired differently is true, but recognizing that did not remove my irritation when we would be threatened with arriving someplace late, such as a doctor's appointment, even as I surely recognized, once in the doctor's office we would no doubt have to wait to be seen. That didn't matter to me. I just wanted to hold up my end of the arrangement by arriving on time.

In a similar way, I always know what day it is. I know when to expect money to arrive, or when an obligation must be paid, and keep those two in balance with each other. True, I now use the calendar on my phone to check my memory, but most of the time that is unnecessary.

But now, that clarity, that orderliness is undercut by the uncertainty of our situation. On my desk in my office is that ancient manually controlled perpetual calendar I've described before. Its display of day and date has to be changed by hand each day. For years, for as long as I have owned that little device, and we're talking about something I have had for close to half a century, long before digital calendars, I scrupulously changed the day and date on it.

However, a year ago in August I let it stay on the twelfth of that month, marking the day without conscious intent when we stopped going upstairs to our bedroom. Tracy reminded me, when I mentioned this date, that it is grandson Evan's birthday. With all due respect to Evan, the more immediate significance of that date to this context is the day when we abandoned the effort to have Carol mount the stairs to our bedroom.

That moment is now captured on that device.

Yet, on my office wall and the kitchen wall are two 2018 calendars, each kept correctly on the right month. And my new watch correctly shows the date every day.

Thus, the contradiction.

Emblematic in some way of my unsettled mind, my present ambivalence to time, that erstwhile rock-solid constant in my relationship to the world.

Tracy's group message drew me in, with some force, to the present.

Yet that present still seems to me to be somehow unreal as I try without much success to wrap my mind around where we now are.

Note 1: After some back and forth regarding its last line, my story "Like Water Over Stones" was accepted by Rosebud.

Note 2: The Toyota representative did call to tell me that the Pandora problem was going to be fixed in November by removing that app from the Entune Suite.

A Scare

Monday night after dinner. Carol still in her chair after eating at the dining room table. Soon I will want to move her into her bed for the night, so I am stealing a few minutes of writing time now. A little later I will be watching the late Dodgers game from the coast.

This morning as we were both rousing, Carol clearly called out "Steve."

I answered, "I am right here on the couch."

She replied, "I know."

What exactly did she know? That I was where I said I was? That is the minimum, I suppose, acknowledging that my male voice came from close by. That I was the one always nearby? To be sure.

But what about the next step, and the one after it? First that I was Steve, and, here's the important part, the Steve who is her husband, is now her husband and not was her husband as a shard of memory.

Of course, even the minimum answer is a positive, showing her connection to the here and now as she woke up. The moving up the scale toward her acknowledging me as her present mate is maddening.

Maddening because it makes the present unclear and the future uncertain. I do not think that the downward course of this disease can be changed. Perhaps stabilized for a while. But for how long?

I am so used to thinking in known time intervals, so many days before the third Wednesday when my Social Security check is deposited, or years ago, charting when I would retire, the timing of life's moments big and small, has always been clear to me.

But not now.

I don't know if I would be happier with a timetable telling me how this disease is going to work itself out.

Sort of like the clichéd question asking what would you do, if you had 24 hours to live as a matter of certainty.

A timetable would provide the kind of certainty I am used to dealing with.

But the point is, I don't want this damned disease to complete its job.

Thursday night. No music on. Trying to squeeze out some words. There are times, fortunately for me not very often, when I have to push hard to get started, when the blank screen and the beckoning keys do not perform their usual magic of opening up that part of my brain from which language, almost unbidden, usually flows.

So, we'll start and see what happens.

Today, Clare, the nurse practitioner, gave Carol a good report on her physical condition. Beyond that she shared what has now been a repeated observation that Carol seems more aware, more responsive, and less resistant, all good signs. Clare asked if Carol ever smiled.

"Yes," I said, "on occasion."

"Are you familiar with FAST?" Clare asked.

"No."

She tapped the keys on her notebook and brought up a screen with that acronym as its heading. Below the heading was a list of the seven stages of dementia. Next to number seven was the notation of losing the ability to smile. Apparently, FAST is a dementia scale, a tool that indicates the degree the disease has reached.

Clearly, I was not happy that Clare's question about smiling appears on the end of the scale.

"Does that make you uncomfortable?" she asked.

"Yes," I replied. "But with or without it, I know what I am dealing with."

We turned in a more positive direction.

"We can increase the dosage of galantamine," she said,

"assuming it is responsible for the improvements in Carol's condition."

And so we agreed to up the dose from sixteen mg a day to twenty-four, the maximum allowable. Perhaps the increased dosage of this medicine, which Carol has only been on for a few months, will continue the improvement.

I am doubtful.

Well, some words came, and now it is time for sleep. Tomorrow I intend to go to the main library in town for another writing session.

When I arrived home from the library in town yesterday, Tonda, the aide, was apologetic. "I could not get her to eat lunch," she said. "I tried, but she just went back to sleep and has been sleeping all afternoon."

I assured Tonda that this was not that unusual. Carol often slept a lot in the afternoon and was not always interested in lunch.

True.

But I was mistaken.

After Tonda left, I could not rouse Carol for more than a few seconds. She felt a little warm to me. But Tonda had said that Carol had complained about being chilled and so she had bundled her under two blankets. I removed one. After a while, she remained warm to my touch. I was able to rouse her a little bit, long enough for her to sip some water, and take one apathetic bite of a protein bar.

And then back to sleep.

Suppertime was approaching. Carol seemed to be drooling a little bit. I wasn't sure her eyes were focusing properly.

Was she having, or had she had, a seizure?

I tried talking to her, but she did not respond.

I was getting seriously worried.

What to do?

It was late afternoon, after five, but I called Chronic Care anyway. Predictably I got a message that the office was closed.

But at the end of the message, there were instructions for help with a medical condition that could not wait. Call Munson Hospital and ask for the Chronic Care provider on call to be paged.

I did.

Within a few minutes, the phone rang. My caller ID indicated "Private Caller."

Just what I need, I thought. A junk call. I don't always let the answering machine take those calls because the caller often leaves thirty or so seconds of static. I pick up the phone as though answering it and then hang it up.

But this time before I could get to the phone the answering machine had been activated and I heard a voice identifying herself as the on-duty Chronic Care provider.

Much relieved, I spoke with Angela. I described what I had been dealing with, speculated that maybe Carol had come down with something that produced a fever, didn't think, as I was giving voice to thoughts running through my head, that she had had a stroke because she had been able to squeeze my hand. Yes, Angela replied, that sounds right. A seizure? Possibly, if she had already had one it would be hard to tell. I would like to check her temperature, I said, but I won't be able to get her to hold the thermometer in her mouth.

"Hold it under her armpit," Angela replied.

"Oh?"

"Yes. It'll take a little longer to get a reading, and it'll be about a degree lower."

I looked over at Carol at the short-sleeved nightshirt she was wearing, contemplating having to remove that.

"That'll be a bit of a process," I said.

"Well, keep an eye on her. What time do you usually have supper?"

"About seven, seven-thirty."

"See if you can rouse her to eat something," she said.

But as that time approached, and she still felt warm, and unresponsive, I called again.

"I'm going to try to take her temperature," I told Angela.

I did not try to remove the nightshirt. Instead, I rolled up the short sleeve far enough for me to get the bulb of the thermometer nestled in her armpit and held it there. When I thought I had held it there long enough, I took it out.

It read 100.

Add 1. 101.

I wanted to be sure it had been under her arm long enough, so I put it back for another minute, removed it, read it.

Still 100.

I reported the result to Angela.

"Shall I give her aspirin?" I asked.

"Tylenol would be better," she replied.

In the downstairs bathroom there was Motrin but no Tylenol. I still had the phone in my hand and told Angela I was going to look in the upstairs bathroom.

I did and found Tylenol.

"How much?" I asked.

"Is it tablets or capsules?"

"Tablets."

"One and a half. Can you cut one?"

"I have a pill splitter," I replied.

I administered that dosage in applesauce, as I give Carol all her meds.

In about an hour, the phone rang. It was Angela.

"I'm about to check her temperature," I said.

"I'll wait on the line," she said.

This time the thermometer read 97. Add 1. 98.

"Good," Angela said. "Try to give her some supper. Call me if you need to. I'm on all night."

Carol roused, and ate some yogurt, drank some water.

Went back to sleep.

I fixed myself a frozen dinner.

This morning, the phone rang again. I don't recall what the caller ID said. I answered it. It was another nurse from Munson. I told her Carol now seemed okay.

And she was.

She had a full breakfast and a good lunch. No sign of fever. I expect she will eat her supper in a while.

That's what happened. I still need to digest and then write about it.

Perhaps tomorrow.

A Cold Winter Ahead

Thursday night. Classical music from WSHU in my earbuds. Carol in bed, but not yet fully asleep. She breathes loudly through her mouth. I imagine her nose is stuffed. Nothing I can do about that.

And the sound reasserts her presence.

It's been almost a week since last Friday when I came home to find Carol ill. She has been better since then, but the incident has awakened concerns I have been keeping at bay, but which now insist on being addressed.

There are two such, intimately related and one or the other will happen: either Carol will predecease me, or I her. I've dealt with the second by setting up a trust, but not in the manner in which it might occur. That is for another time.

The first, which I confront now, involves the prospect of my living alone into old age.

Some people experience a version of living alone as young adults moving out into their own apartment either when getting a full-time job or even renting a place while in college as an alternative to dorm living.

I did neither. I attended a college about a mile from my house and across the street from my high school to which I had walked rather than take the bus. I spent my undergraduate years in my parents' house, first walking and later occasionally driving my '52 Packard to college. In graduate school at the University of Connecticut, I lived in a private room in a dorm. That was a small step toward living alone. Then I married.

It was when that marriage ended that I fully set up housekeeping for myself, renting an apartment and furnishing it with second-hand pieces bought from a colleague who had gone through his own divorce and had the furniture in storage. I still needed a bed so working in my college's theater shop, I built a platform variety of one with a bookcase for a headboard.

So, I was now living alone. It did not seem difficult because in many ways my life went on in its usual fashion. I went to my job as a professor and administrator. Part of my old married life continued into my single condition as on alternate weekends I had my two daughters with me.

Of course, this was a difficult, stressful time because of the impending divorce, but I didn't fret about my solitary status. I was still relatively young. My life lay ahead of me and I was going to reinvent myself in my relationship with Carol who soon became the center of all else that whirled around me.

And I was still rooted in New York among friends, colleagues, familiar geography and close to my daughters as they grew up.

After a while, Carol and I lived together, then married after my divorce was finalized and my solo living ended.

Now, however, it is possible that I might find myself in my twilight years living alone in northern Michigan, a thousand miles from what I've left behind in New York: two daughters and grandchildren, as well as several very long-term friends. It is also likely that my daughter with Carol, who is now living six hundred miles away in Minnesota, will wind up someplace other than here. And although I have lived here for sixteen years, my roots in this foreign territory are still quite shallow, the friendships I have made not yet fully matured. All in all, a very different set of circumstances than I experienced long ago.

A chance encounter put this speculation into focus for me.

The other day I ran into a neighbor on the checkout line in the grocery in town. My relationship with him falls somewhere between an acquaintance on the one hand and a friend on the other. Like Carol, his family has been on this peninsula for a very long time although more as hoteliers than farmers.

We chatted a little. I asked him what his plans were for the winter, a pretty standard topic of conversation hereabout as our winters are long and difficult. The local population divides into those who head to warmer climes for the whole season, those who leave for a few weeks, and those who stay the whole time. Carol and I fluctuated between the second and third categories, occasionally traveling to Florida for a break from the snow and cold.

He said he planned on going to Texas to visit a friend, and then to Oregon to spend time with his son.

Why this conversation was more than social chatter for me is that he is roughly in my age group, perhaps a little younger. His background is, I believe, in psychology, perhaps as a counselor or therapist. He is also an accomplished painter whose works hang in the gallery attached to the tavern up the road from here. He's a good enough handyman to maintain his family's rental cottages, he is something of a sailor, and also has a second place in town.

None of which is why I am talking about him.

Rather, I see in him what I might become down the road, living here as a single older man.

In that respect his travel plans for the upcoming winter indicate the freedom of movement such a person enjoys as opposed to the limits on my movements imposed upon me by my caregiving responsibilities. The question in my mind is whether *enjoys* is an accurate word to attach to my expectation that I, too, might be as free as he appears to be to deal with the winter as he likes, and more generally, to do what he wants to do when he wants to do it.

Having now years of experience in northern Michigan, I imagine living a solitary existence on this snowbound peninsula with the winds howling in off the waters of the bay and through the less than perfect seals of this old farmhouse would be challenging if not depressing. So, perhaps should I find myself in that circumstance, I would also travel to visit children and grandchildren or a very good friend at whose wedding I was his best man, a friend who happens to live in snow-free Florida. In warmer weather, I could visit another good friend now in Syracuse, or ones back on Long Island, or even an older friend who lived across the street from me in Brooklyn and is also in upstate New York in Utica.

At this point, however, hearing Carol's heavy sleep breathing not ten feet away, I cannot even begin to tolerate that thought.

I do not know my neighbor's story, how he came to be an older single man. He does not appear to be at all unhappy with his life. Perhaps he is in a relationship, but I don't know enough about him to begin to guess about that.

It might be worth talking to him at some point.

But not now. It is too damned distressing.

Two Minus One Still Equals Two

Wednesday evening after a freakish weather day, more like mid-summer with a thunderstorm and winds, and another storm brewing outside. We had a good, quiet day in spite of the weather, of which Carol seemed unaware.

On Saturday, when it was clear that whatever had caused Carol's fever the day before was gone, I went downstairs to the furnace room to do my half hour on the treadmill. Because I am not in great shape, although improving as a result of my new regimen, I strain a bit during the exercise.

On this occasion, when I was breathing a little harder, a morbid thought occurred to me. What if I had a fatal heart attack? That thought presented itself in a particularly vivid way. I imagined myself lying dead on the treadmill, the machine still running, my body jammed against the machine's stanchions.

For three days.

While upstairs in the living room Carol would be in her hospital bed unattended.

Because as I live now, from Friday afternoon when my relief aide leaves until Tuesday afternoon when next an aide arrives, I rarely have interaction with anybody. Except for telemarketers of one sort or another, the phone does not ring. Nobody drops by. Any contact I have during this period occurs because I initiated it. I do go to the market every Sunday morning and at least one of the clerks there as well as the manager, is well aware of these habitual visits to pick up a muffin for Carol and the *Times* if it is available, but I doubt that familiarity would alarm either of them if I did not show up.

I shared this concern with my daughter Tracy. She said she would make it her business to call every weekend to make sure I was still among the living.

I also talked about this concern with my lunch companions. Brad suggested a digital approach: scheduling an automatic email arriving in my inbox, to which I would respond. Probably a better strategy than Tracy's regular call. She could set up the recurring email and check her inbox for my response.

Enough morbidity for one night.

Carol breathing very heavily in her sleep.

I enjoy the sound.

Late Sunday afternoon. Sitting in the green room, having just watched a football game. Carol asleep in her bed in the living room, the radio still tuned to the classical music from Interlochen Public Radio. In an hour or so, I'll prepare supper. Then, I'll be back in this room for Sunday night television.

Tonight, I'll watch a new season of Poldark *on* Masterpiece. *Like most of these productions it is high-class soap made a bit more substantial by its historical setting. More relevant to me now and what I am about to explore is the recurrent sadness I still experience in watching these shows alone. In fact, it is not unlikely that I continue to make sure I watch them as a way of preserving a piece of our shared life together, as we always, that is always, watched the PBS shows on Sunday night.*

There are two green reclining chairs in this room.

I sit in the one closest to the window wall, the one on the left if I am facing the television.

Carol always sat in the chair on the right.

While watching the game I worked the Sunday crossword puzzle on my laptop during the frequent time-outs and halftime. As I did, at a certain point, my laptop, which was running on battery, warned me that I needed to find another power source.

I retrieved its power cord from the living room and plugged

it in to the outlet on the wall nearest Carol's chair. The cord was long enough for me to sit back down in my chair

Which I did.

I would not sit in Carol's chair. To do so would be unthinkable.

How so?

It would make sense not to stretch the power cord across the floor any farther than necessary. But to sit in Carol's chair would confirm the obvious fact that never again will she sit in it. Of course, that is true. I just don't want to confirm it to myself. It is one of many instances where I face the same situation, namely, how to deal with the lingering facts of how we shared space in this house.

Of course, there are features in the house that cannot easily be changed, such as the his and hers bookcases attached to the dining room wall. Or her dresser across from mine in our bedroom. Or her office down the hall from mine.

And so on.

In ways large and small, our living space announces that is serves two people.

To this point, I am content to leave it that way.

I've moved into the living room to sit in my usual chair. Our sofa is in this room but there is only one chair, Steve's chair, which Carol ordered for me along with a reading lamp to stand beside it. I don't believe Carol ever sat in it. Across from me now, though, is her new chair, the tilt wheelchair in which she spends a good chunk of her waking, and not so waking, hours during the day. To my left is the hospital bed on which she is now rousing from her afternoon nap.

On my way into the living room I stopped in the kitchen to grab a handful of peanuts for a snack. While in the kitchen locating the peanut jar in the cabinet over the stove, I was reminded that the shelves in another section of this cabinet were filled with boxes of tea, all kinds of tea, mostly herbal, designed to be a natural cure for various conditions having to do with digestion, as Carol's stomach was troublesome, and these teas, all of them, are hers.

Very occasionally I feel like having a cup of tea, perhaps as memory reminds me how my father, following his English heritage, drank tea with supper. He, of course, would not abide tea bags. His tea had to be brewed from tea leaves. I'll use tea bags for mine, and among Carol's medicinal teas is her Earl Grey's.

Put simply. I drink coffee, rarely tea. Carol never drank coffee, which unsettled her stomach, and therefore drank tea.

Tea and coffee.

Carol and Steve.

Sharing space in this house.

Even now.

Although Carol is more like a living memory of herself.

Which I intend to hold onto.

Until perhaps all traces are gone.

What's in a Name and a Squeeze
of the Hand

*Monday night. Ryan came by for dinner and I retrieved
a pizza from town. Carol, as usual, enjoyed a couple of
slices although I reminded her this pizza was not from our
beloved Papa Nick's back on Long Island.*

This morning at breakfast, Carol stopped chewing the
piece of toast I had just given her and said quite distinctly,
"Steve."

Nothing more. Just my name.

I assured her that I was sitting right next to her as always.
She finished chewing.

What to make of this one word, said with so much emphasis.

First, she does not articulate words clearly very often.
When she does it is usually because she is upset about something when she might say "Stop" or just simply "No." Those
words uttered clearly and with emphasis. Occasionally, she
forms other words, such as "yes" or more rarely a whole
short sentence, such as "I like that," although that last is
quite infrequent.

She does talk a fair amount by which I mean she makes
sounds in which it is difficult to find recognizable words.

I recognize that losing the power to articulate words is a
predictable result of her disease.

None of which brings me any closer to dealing with what
she said this morning other than it was an example of a
clearly articulated word.

Which happens to be my name.

When I was sitting not two feet away from her.

But to what purpose? And from what storehouse in her
brain was it recovered?

I permit myself to let my spirits be raised by hearing my
name coming out of her mouth. But I also recognize that it

is important not to put too much weight on the event. Perhaps the word is no more than a shard of long-term memory. Even so, why give it voice? It was not said in a tone that revealed its intent. I can't say she was troubled and looking for help from that ancient source, the bit of her husband remaining in her brain.

In fact, when well she rarely if ever asked for my help in anything. She was too damned independent and self-sufficient. She was more likely to offer to help me.

Has that changed?

Does she now in the throes of her illness feel she needs help? That possibility pulls at my heart as sometimes a certain expression on her face does as well when that expression seems to indicate if not fear then maybe confusion or sadness. Or maybe frustration in the recognition of what she can no longer do, she who thought that through an exercise of her indomitable will she could do anything. She did overcome her fear of public speaking so that in law school she could perform in moot court; she overcame her fear of flying by, well, just boarding the plane.

I know I am overanalyzing this one-word utterance of my name.

And I haven't even addressed the perplexing question as to whether she associates that name with present tense me. Of course, I'd like to think so, but I don't want to be foolish about it.

And there is no certainty about any of this, just speculation.

Which I will be well-advised to understand is just that.

I don't even know what certainty I would prefer because any conclusion that can be drawn would offer a mixture of pain and comfort.

Comfort in suggesting we are still in some fashion together, a pale echo of what once we were.

And pain in both the recognition of that paleness and the reminder of what has been lost if this crumb, this utterance, is all that is left.

Tuesday night after my usual shopping day. Tired, but I

want to capture what just occurred, which is a continuation of what I wrote last session.

Carol is now asleep. I did a simple thing with her I had not done before.

I held her hand as she fell asleep.

I routinely hold her hand at various times during the day. I enjoy the physical contact, which approximates in a faint kind of way the intimacy we used to have, the comfort we enjoyed in each other's physical closeness.

Typically, when I take Carol's hand, she seems to squeeze mine. Sometimes, perhaps, I have tightened my grip on her hand, but other times she acts first. I do not know if this is a neurological response devoid of any conscious intention. And her grip can be quite strong in such moments so that I need to exert a little effort to free my hand.

I'd like to think, however, that there is intention in that squeeze of the hand, that she wants to feel my flesh against her, that it provides her some comfort. At other times when I clasp her hand, she brings her other hand on top of mine. Again, I cannot be sure of intention if any for often enough she holds her own hands together perhaps as a way of staying their wayward motion.

That perplexed and perplexing preface brings me to tonight.

After I had her settled in her bed, I took her hand. As so many times before she closed her fingers around mine and then added her other hand.

I did not pull my hand away after a few moments as I ordinarily would. Instead, I studied her face, which seemed to relax. Then her eyes closed. Her breathing moved into its sleeping rhythm.

I waited a bit more. Then very carefully, so as not to disturb her, I slipped my hand out of her grasp.

She did not waken.

As with her calling my name, I cannot with any certainty analyze this occurrence.

Whatever the actuality, I will assume some level of conscious intention, or if not intention awareness and contentment that I was there in physical contact with her.

Perhaps it is foolish to have such thoughts.

But if so, I don't care.

Because whatever its source, with or without conscious intention or deliberate response, just like hearing my name in her voice, these seemingly insignificant instances are my reward, the sustenance that .feeds my determination to stay the course.

If this is what my job is now, and my pay, so be it.

Note: Both halves of my two-part heading to this entry are literary allusions. First Shakespeare, then Melville.

I couldn't help myself.

No Surrender

After midnight Sunday night. I have been busy the past few days working on my new writing opportunity as a columnist for the local newspaper. It is important for me so to do to maintain the semblance of balance in my life. The result, though, is I haven't had as much time or energy for this project, and it is too late to do much tonight.

I'll scratch out a few words in the hope I can pick up some momentum tomorrow.

As usual I watched PBS tonight, first *Poldark* and then a documentary on Itzhak Perlman. Nothing unusual in that fact. What was different was that Carol, in her chair, was in the TV room with me. Not in her bed. Or drowsing in her chair in the living room. But in her chair a few feet away from me, positioned in front of the recliner in which she would sit when we watched television together.

I did not come to the decision to wheel her into this room this evening lightly. I don't want to overanalyze this, but it is worth a little exploration. I was happy to have her in the room with me even though, for the most part, she was asleep. I say for the most part because at least once she laughed at something humorous in the Perlman piece. So maybe she was drifting in and out of sleep and processing, as she does, what she hears rather than what she sees. At any rate, I don't now recall what she found funny, but I am sure that her laugh was in response to the audio from the show, and not from a voice in her head.

I guess having her in the room with me, in front of her own chair, can be seen as an effort on my part to hold onto a piece of our pre-disease lives. I don't see anything wrong with that when there really is no better alternative in our situation. When, as usual, I watch television alone while she dozes in her chair in the living room until it is time to transfer to her bed, that separation is a concession to her disease that might ultimately prevail.

But not just yet. Her presence in the TV room in front of her chair, occasionally responding to some bit of audio is a useful fiction that I intend to continue as a retention of the past because that past unexpectedly recurs from time to time.

Such as this morning when I was in the kitchen beginning to prepare breakfast when from her bed, I heard her call, quite distinctly, my name. I called "What?" to her.

I didn't expect her to respond, and she didn't.

But that brief interaction had the feel of our old-time normalcy.

"I'm fixing breakfast," I continued.

As I would have done in the past. Perhaps she heard and processed what I said. I can never be sure. Often when I leave her for a little while such as to run down to the store or the post office, or even across the road to get the mail, I tell her what I am doing, ask if it is okay, and when I return I tease her by asking if she has missed me.

And fairly often she says yes.

So, I continue to hold up my end of the conversational possibilities and am rewarded when she picks up her end. It is well worth doing, not only for her occasional response but for my own head, a way to combat the strong sense that I am living alone.

Wednesday night. A few snow showers mixed in with rain announce the approach of winter. A little snow remained on the ground for some hours. My snowblower is repaired and ready. Am I?

At my weekly lunch last Thursday, on an impulse, perhaps suggested by Carol's recent, robust appetite for lunch wherein she happily ate a grilled cheese sandwich, in addition to ordering my usual wrap, I requested a half wrap for Carol. I always used to get two wraps for when I was picking up lunch for us. I did this so regularly that I just had to identify myself when I called and say I was coming by to pick up our usual sandwiches and they would be waiting for me. As Carol's disease progressed, a whole wrap began to be more than she wanted, and so I would get her a half. But the ingredients for each remained the same, turkey in mine, ham in hers, lettuce and tomato in both, mayo in mine, Thousand Island dressing and black olives in hers.

Then, even that seemed more than she wanted, and I stopped getting her one.

Until this past Thursday when I ordered one for her, asking Ardie, who runs the place, whether I was right in remembering that when Carol was still eating her wraps she had given up on black olives.

"Yes," Ardie answered. "That's right."

So I took her half wrap home, and put it in the refrigerator for another time because the aide had already given Carol lunch.

I look for reasons to avoid cooking full meals seven days a week, so on Friday, reviving an old pattern, I heat up chicken noodle soup from a can, add toast for Carol and a PBJ sandwich for me. I had intended this time to substitute the wrap for her toast, but I forgot.

Until Saturday when I remembered the wrap in the refrigerator and offered it to Carol for lunch.

She devoured it with enthusiasm.

So, our new/old normal for now and for as long as it lasts, will include a weekly half wrap for Carol.

It is a little thing, it seems, but a little thing of some importance. In so many ways, large and small, our lives teeter between what was and what will be, and the best we can do is try to find stasis between those two conditions. And in that stasis whatever presents itself as a continuation of the old into our new present is welcome whereas any adjustment that denies the possibility of what used to be continuing is most unwelcome.

Perhaps all of that sounds like too much weight to put on a half wrap containing ham, lettuce, tomato, and Thousand Island dressing sans black olives.

But I don't think so.

And I might even push a little further. I used to add one of the wonderful, freshly baked cookies to go along with Carol's wrap. I still always get one with mine.

So, this next time, I'll go for it, and get one for her.

This stubborn retention of bits of our past is an act of resistance to push back against the power of dementia to eradicate that past.

The alternative is surrender and I don't see us doing that any time soon.

The Necessity of Routine

Late Sunday night, too late to start anything of substance, so I'll just mention a couple of things, and then see what I can do tomorrow.

Thing one: A little while ago I held Carol's hand as she fell asleep. I have been doing that regularly, and perhaps will have more to say about it.

Thing two: I ordered Carol's half wrap at lunch on Friday and served it to her that evening with our regular chicken soup plus sandwich dinner. The sandwich used to be tuna fish. She ate the wrap with enthusiasm.

Monday night after a pretty good day. Cleaners came so house is in better shape, and Ryan joined us for a Chinese take-out dinner. He'll stop by tomorrow to give me a hand hauling up the heavy storm doors as it's time to get serious about the oncoming winter.

The main plus today at the end of my long weekend is an opportunity for social interaction and conversation with both the cleaners, who have been coming here for years, and, of course, Ryan. I need to find ways to combat isolation, so as to build on these people interactions. I am planning on using respite time later in the week to go to town to see a movie, probably the new Redford one. Maybe even stumble into somebody I know.

Over the weekend Tracy called on Saturday and Danielle texted me on Sunday, and those contacts seem to be becoming regular occurrences. That eases my mind about the long hiatus each weekend when nobody would know if I were alive or dead. Not a morbid thought, just a practical one.

I read in today's newspaper how a woman was stuck in her bathtub for five days because she couldn't reach a grab bar. She used warm water for heat and drank cold water for five days until a mail carrier noticed her mail accumulating and that discovery led to her being rescued from her predicament.

So not morbid, just practical.

That issue shelved for the while, it looks like our lives have settled in to a potentially long, stable period. Carol's cognitive issues, if anything, are a touch better, and her physical health remains good. She is eating well. Her nose still is stuffed as is mine, but she is not having much difficulty swallowing.

I am a creature of habit and function best within routine, and that is where I am now. Our daily pattern does not vary much. In the morning, I transfer Carol to her chair and into the kitchen for breakfast; then we move back into the living room where she dozes in her chair, and I do puzzles, or write or attend to correspondence on my laptop; lunch follows for both of us, Carol sometimes still in her chair, other times in bed while I generally eat mine in the kitchen; after lunch on non-respite relief days we follow the routine very much like the mornings with Carol back in her bed after a while in her chair while I again get on my laptop for work, socialization, or amusement; for supper Carol is in her chair at the dining room table; after supper, she remains in her chair while I watch a little television and after a couple of hours transfer Carol back to her bed; later, usually about eleven, I get her ready for sleep, and once she is settled, I follow my lifelong habit of writing in a silent house. Then, I read for a while lying on the couch where I sleep. Some time ago, I bought a wrap around your neck reading device with two small bulbs that produce concentrated beams sufficient to illuminate the pages of a book. Using it, I can read while the rest of the room remains dark. Reading before I sleep is another old habit.

Thus, the rhythm of our lives in a comfortable, repetitive pattern. I, of course, still often feel isolated, legitimately so, but the routine is a great help.

For both of us.

I believe Carol has responded well to the patterning of our lives. I don't know, absent any research, whether such patterning is thought to be good for dementia patients, but my observation would suggest it is.

The one moment in this routine that is new and which I most deeply appreciate is my holding hands with Carol as she falls to sleep. It is now a regular part of our routine. I sit on the edge of her bed and take her hand. She returns the pressure, and usually places her other hand on top of mine.

I treasure these moments as I sit next to her, feeling the pressure of her fingers around mine, and studying her face as her breathing becomes regular and she relaxes into sleep. When I am sure she is fully asleep, I remove my hand from her grip as gently as possible, stand up, and turn off the lamp that is behind her bed.

It is a pale echo of how we used to sleep together, but it still provides a sense of physical intimacy that transient as it is, as much as a reminder of a lost past as it is, puts a gentle close to my caregiving responsibilities.

Then, since it is usually not yet midnight, and my biorhythm perks up at that time, I write.

As I have always done.

This ordering of our lives, into which I mix the necessary chores of keeping food in the house, paying bills, attending to whatever problems the house, inside and out, decides to present, schedule necessary doctor appointments for both of us, this structure enables me to maintain my equanimity in the face of this most difficult situation.

And it does one more thing, a most necessary thing: it provides regularly recurring time slots during which I can write, as well as to attend to the business end of writing. I don't have as much time, or energy for that matter, as perhaps I once did. But what I have is enough for me to continue practicing what is so essential to my nature.

Were she able, I am sure Carol would agree as she was always so supportive of me in that regard.

Were I to stop, I believe I would be failing both of us.

Anyway, I don't think I could if I wanted to.

At the Movies

Carol is sleeping noisily, her mouth open. The dog is asleep on the floor. My energy is fading so I think I will join them in slumber after I lay out a thread to be continued.

At lunch with my friends some time ago, the conversation turned to movies recently watched. I felt a little envious and mentioned I hadn't been to see a film since Carol's illness became serious, now about two years ago.

"Why don't you use one of your respite afternoons?" somebody suggested.

Why not indeed?

I go shopping on one respite afternoon, have lunch out on another, and the third is available for necessary appointments, but also for unplanned, or out of the ordinary events.

Such as going to a movie.

Which I would do alone. And that gave me pause.

One of the things I look to do during my respite times is to interact with other people since my life is otherwise so confined to me, Carol, and the dog.

So I have my weekly lunch with my guys, and occasionally when I have time after some other errand I will have a sandwich at the old general store where I can chat with Marci and provide an audience for Jim's endless barrel of tales, many of them of the tall variety.

A solo movie trip would be different. I am alone when I shop. But that is a chore and involves movement and interaction. It's true that Carol and I always food shopped together, but I recall eons ago in my first marriage occasionally doing the weekly grocery shopping by myself because doing so happened to fit better into our working schedules.

So doing that now does not feel at all odd.

In a similar fashion, I usually went to my doctor appointments alone as did Carol before she could no longer manage to do that.

But what I had not done as far back as I can remember is go to the movies alone. We always went together.

That's the point, of course, we did enjoyable things together.

After a lifetime lived one way, this new idea of attending a movie by myself is both exciting and off-putting. I guess those competing feelings make a certain amount of sense.

Off-putting because I almost feel I am abandoning Carol to indulge myself in an experience she cannot share. I realize by any rational standard that is a ridiculous thought. It is, after all, my respite time. I should be doing something I enjoy. That is the point of respite time. I do have these three time slots each week when I can leave the house and know Carol is being well attended.

Up until now, I have used these slots for purposes that felt necessary and/or right: shopping, lunch with friends, and occasionally work, as in a writing session in the library.

But never in these two years, have I done something for my amusement alone. In fact, I cannot recall throughout my whole life ever going to any kind of amusement, be it a film, a concert, a sports event, alone. I may have, but none come to mind.

That recognition explains why the thought of going to this movie by myself offers an element of excitement. It will be something new. There is the outside possibility that I might bump into somebody I know. But more interesting is seeing the world, for a brief period, as an unattached free agent.

Of course, I know that at the deepest level, I dread that state. But it will be interesting to experience it for a couple of hours before sliding back into the now very familiar patterns of my caregiving responsibilities.

And so I will embark on this embarrassingly trivial adventure and see how it goes.

Thursday night, after midnight, jazz from KNKX in my earbuds.

This afternoon during my respite time I drove into town, parked my car in the public garage. Walking from the parking garage to the theater did not seem right. In downtown Traverse City on an avenue lined with restaurants and shops, almost everybody else was walking with someone.

Walking and talking.

The only solitary walkers, like myself, seemed to be moving faster as if they were late for an appointment.

Or like me, they had no one with whom to share whatever it was they were doing, whether shopping, or dining, or attending to some kind of business.

I found myself picking up my pace to match theirs, even though I was not at all late for the start of the film, which in any event would be preceded by ten or fifteen minutes of coming attractions.

That short walk thrust me into life without Carol. A small part of me felt a little curiosity, a mix of apprehension but also a bit of excitement as though turning the page into a new chapter.

Having reached the State Theater, I bought one ticket for Redford in *The Old Man & the Gun*, walked directly in to the candy counter, which seemed a necessary first stop, bought a big bag of M&M's, corrected the change the volunteer gave me, and then strolled through the doors into the cavernous seating area of this renovated building to a seat in the middle of an otherwise empty row, and settled down, feeling quite strange.

The sparse members of the audience scattered at significant distances from each other intensified the strangeness. Redford is an icon, the movie got pretty good reviews, and although this was a weekday afternoon showing, I had expected a larger crowd. In a more usual movie viewing experience I would be aware, even without conversation, of those around me. Watching a movie in a theater is essentially a communal affair. That is part of the fun.

I was engrossed in the film as I would have been had Carol been sitting by my side. As I usually do, I followed the plot and tried to anticipate how it would end. Would the screenwriters succeed in that difficult task of providing a satisfying conclusion, one that seemed both plausible and meaningful in terms created by the plot? I imagine other writers of fiction who spend inordinate amounts of time constructing narratives that carry the reader to a good conclusion might also view film narratives this way. I do pay attention, of course, to the visual elements of film and the acting. But for me narrative construction is primary.

I was not entirely pleased with this film's ending, but I conceded that given its plot centered on a career criminal's life alternating between heists and imprisonments from which he would escape, spiced by a late life romance, it would be difficult to do much better.

Back onto the street, I hastened to the parking garage. I had reason to hurry now because I was nearing the end of my respite time. I had told the aide I might run a little late, but I didn't want to abuse the privilege.

In the car, almost without thinking I turned for a moment toward the seat where Carol would be sitting to ask her what she thought of the film.

We always shared out responses, not always agreeing, of course, but happy for the opportunity to bounce our reactions off each other. Often a good conversation would fill up most of the time on the way home.

I turned on the radio and let music fill the vacuum.

Me and Me

Monday night after a pretty good day. Carol laughed more than usual, sometimes at something she heard, sometimes at something humorous in her head. Ryan joined us for a pizza supper, and he noticed the increase in her good humor. And she ate three slices.

Got some positive responses to my second column for the Record-Eagle, *one in which within my 550–600 word limit I attempted to deal with the mystery of the inaccessible thoughts that Carol clearly contemplates in silence, a kind of daydreaming although far more focused than that from the look on her face.*

The responses to my column, and the fact I have undertaken the responsibility of a regular gig writing for the local newspaper leads me into what I have been thinking about which, for want of a better word, I will term the schizophrenia of my life now that Carol has seemingly settled into a stable period, and my caregiving routines are well established so that each day is pretty much laid out for me in terms of what I have to do and what space is available for things I might want to do.

Prominent in the latter category is my life as a writer.

I have always found time to write, no matter what else was going on in my life, what other responsibilities demanded my attention, or bright shiny object lured me away. Maybe that is why I almost always write late at night when the house is quiet and all chores have been attended to, and distractions would have to be sought.

Or maybe it is just a matter of my natural biorhythm favoring that time frame right before sleep. In any case, from day to day I must be writing on something.

So that is the schizophrenia I am talking about. Of course,

I am using the term metaphorically to suggest that I am, in a certain sense, two people.

I am Carol's caregiver having assumed those responsibilities thrust upon me by Carol's disease, a burden I quite willingly have undertaken in spite of the demands, emotional and physical, that it places upon me.

And the other me insists on reasserting itself by retaining the interests and activities that have always been constants in my life.

Pausing now having set up this dichotomy to let these thoughts percolate for a while before attempting to flesh them out.

Tuesday night. Sat on the edge of Carol's bed holding her hands with my left hand while with my right I stroked the head of the dog who had come by for her share of my attention. Now both are asleep.

That Currier and Ives domestic scene, husband, wife, dog at bedtime, of course, belies the complexity of our situation. But it is a moment of calm if not serenity, and a good way to end the day.

So I will leave it there for now.

Wednesday night after a Halloween day during which, predictably, no trick or treaters came to the door. We are too far out of town and there are simply no kids around here, hardly anybody much under sixty. Just in case, I had bought a bag of small Three Musketeers, which I have begun to share with Carol.

I've been exploring the idea of the two of me, the one who takes care of Carol, and also runs the household, something we used to share, and the other me with my carryover interests and aspirations. Among the latter is my writing career, which I have been at for about half a century and am not about to give it up now.

As for the first, as Carol's caregiver, after two years I have become pretty well used to it, and for the most part it is now routine. For her part, she seems to have settled into our routine as I have. Most activities go smoothly. She still, as she did earlier this evening, calls my name, and I assured her, as I always do, that I was right there. I continue not to know for a certainty whether she equates my physical presence with my name.

But my name, and associated memories are stored in her brain, and provides me some comfort, small as it is.

I suppose there is a next step when it might become clear that I have in all ways left her memory and at best I will be no more than a figure like anybody else who attends to her needs.

I can't say that I am prepared for the transition to that stage.

As for the carryover Steve, I still read books that interest me, having just finished a slow read of the new biography of Washington Roebling, the engineer who built the Brooklyn Bridge, and will perhaps tonight for a few minutes crack open the next book on my list, Elaine Pagels's study of how Satan evolved from his brief and sometimes not terribly significant appearances in the Old Testament, primarily in the Job story, to his central role in Christianity, including becoming identified with the serpent in the Garden of Eden.

I continue to subscribe to my usual magazines, read the *New York Times* online, do my word puzzles, and follow my sports teams.

Most importantly, I continue to write and keep my writer self visible. Writing a column for the local newspaper gives me an opportunity for regular publication, which most, if not all, writers not only savor but need. Without publication, most give up writing. Others continue, driven perhaps by something like I sense is inside of me, persisting without an audience. I can't say what that something is, perhaps some ego in believing you have something to say, or maybe just the satisfaction of exercising your skill in your craft, as we all enjoy doing what we do well. But whatever it is, publication feeds it.

I think of poor Herman Melville, years after the publication of his *Moby Dick* marked the end of his viability as a published writer, still at his desk, pen in hand, filling the pages of the manuscript that became his wonderful novella *Billy Budd* to be published posthumously thirty-three years later during what became a revival of interest in one of the greatest American fiction writers of his century.

I am not interested in such posthumous fame. And I'll certainly settle for considerably less fame. A little recognition while I am still breathing will do.

So, I still market some of my finished work and I am rewarded every once in a while, as recently I was, with an acceptance, this time of a short story. I have two excellent but as yet unpublished novels waiting for their turn in the spotlight.

I do not think I will have the time or energy for new fiction, at least not in the foreseeable future, and that is too bad.

What is worse about all of this, is that I can no longer share any of it with Carol.

I have to accept that fact. Our relationship wasn't built on our mutual passion for writing. Let's just say it was enhanced by it.

And the solitary version is not nearly as satisfying.

The two of me occupy somewhat uncomfortably the same time and space. At some point one of those two identities will disappear leaving only its memory like tracks in a frozen path that suddenly stops.

Self-Reflection

Thursday afternoon in the community library, where I have not been for some time. As I turned onto the road leading to this building, I passed on that corner the site for the new library, and there I saw that construction had started perhaps trying to get a head start before winter sets in. That new facility will certainly be a boon to our community. The library in its own space will be able to stretch itself with more shelving, a community room for speakers, and so forth. On the downside, perhaps, will be the students at the new charter school now occupying this building will not be able to walk to the library as they now can, and that loss of immediate contact and familiarity with a library is not inconsiderable.

This morning Clare, the nurse practitioner who comes every three weeks or so, checked Carol and found her to be in fine physical shape, and she also remarked on Carol's apparent cognitive improvement.

Which accords with my own observations as well as those of others who have seen Carol over the past weeks.

It seems, then, we have settled into a period of relative stability. As I am a creature of habit, although one who deals with unexpected changes, good or bad, with decent equanimity, I am content to ride this period out for as long as it lasts.

However, on the way out today, Clare asked me if I had plans for a trip to New York in the coming months. She recalled my aborted intent to attend my grandson's bar mitzvah last April, thinking that transporting Carol to the respite facility had turned out to be too expensive but now with her wheelchair, she could more easily, less expensively, be transported in a van supplied with a lift.

Perhaps so. But I explained that travel arrangements, and

the costs thereof, were only part of the problem. My continuing hesitation was emotional, and frankly I don't know if I am ready for a week's separation.

Which I know, on one level, would do me some good.

But on another, I imagine would be difficult.

Would I feel guilty that I was somehow neglecting my responsibilities?

I don't think so because no doubt I would have taken care to be sure Carol would be well attended to in my absence.

Would I think nobody else could replace me?

A ridiculous thought. Three times a week I leave her in the care of my relief aides. True, those times are for only a few hours. Yet, all three aides do a fine job. In that respect, I am eminently replaceable.

But, and this is important, those hours do not include potent emotional periods of going to sleep, rousing in the morning, and in a counterintuitive way, that period of sleep when I lie within a couple of feet of her, when I have held her hand before stretching myself out, and taken her hand upon rising and greeting her in the morning, when during the night I have heard her breathing, or moving about in the bed.

Irrational concerns?

Yes, but who ever said irrational concerns were irrelevant?

Maybe I need to take such a trip once and see how well I and she do. If successful, it can be replicated.

I do need to find out.

But dealing with the impending winter comes first.

Come spring, we will see.

The library is very quiet. I might be the only patron now here. Time to pack up and head home. As I start to close my laptop into its case, I look up and see kids, maybe eight or ten years old, lined up under the supervision of a teacher about to march out of the library and back to their classroom. For all the advantages the new library building will offer, I will miss seeing these young people, their presence surrounded by books somehow suggesting hope for the future.

Monday night before election day. Political robocalls kept my phone ringing with increasing frequency all weekend and into today, the last call arriving well after supper. As usual my caller ID alerted me to these calls and so I didn't bother getting up to answer them. But I noticed that my voice mail was not picking up the calls, and then I remembered the scheduled power outage starting after midnight and into Saturday morning. When the power came back, my answering machine had defaulted to its off position. I switched it back on just in time to catch another call.

That power outage somehow also seemed to have fried the motherboard in my new desktop. At least that is what the Dell tech diagnosed as the reason the unit would not power up. A Dell technician will install a new motherboard on Wednesday, so I've been told.

The falling leaves have opened up my view of East Bay again, a sliver of water more gray than blue now visible. Some trees haven't defoliated yet, so the view will get better in the next week or two.

Which also means that shortly I will be looking out over a blanket of snow as winter is knocking at the door.

It is something over a year since I started keeping this journal and posting weekly blogs from it. I began it for several reasons including sharing my experience both with others in my situation as caregiver, but also all those who are aware of, but have no direct experience with, the growing number of older people sliding into dementia. From a more personal motivation, I need to be writing on something, and this serves that purpose. And finally, as a writer, I always consider publication, and so this material might become a book down the road.

A less obvious consequence of my regular writing about

our situation is that it forces me to think about it rather than just react to it. I believe that is a valuable by-product. Caregiving responsibilities can be exhausting.

But they can also become through repetition rather mindless.

And that is not a good thing.

Not for the recipient of the care, nor the provider of it.

On that reflective note, which had never occurred to me before it just popped into my head, I will close this session with one last thought.

As a writing instructor for many years, I always encouraged students to think of writing as recursive. Reading what one has just written often enough leads to another idea, one that would not have occurred to the writer had he or she not been writing.

It is good to understand that as a writer.

But also, as a tool for the caregiver.

More than writing about our everyday activities, or even the problematic situations that arise and must be handled, when I sit down at my laptop, I open a door into my mind, and perhaps most importantly, my feelings. It makes me more self-reflective than I usually am.

And that, too, is a good thing. That is what in hindsight I see is precisely what I was doing when delving into how I felt, and feel, about taking time off from my caregiving responsibilities.

My wonderfully gifted wife placed a quote attributed to E.M. Forster beneath her email signature. It is an apt closing quote: "How will I know what I think until I see what I say?"

Writing as an act of discovery, as a way to open the door to thoughts and feelings.

New and Newer Normal

Friday night, wind howling outside, snow already on the ground. But at least the phone has stopped ringing, Election Day having come and gone. This is not the place to chew over the results, just glad it's over.

Welcome distraction from all the political noise came from reading the reprint of an article from the 2007 issue of The New York Review of Books. *The article was a review of books about the founding of Jamestown. The reviewer was Edmund Morgan, one of the main secondary sources for my dissertation and I was always immensely impressed not only by his scholarship but the clarity of his prose, a pleasure to read. Reacquainting myself with him was like getting back in touch with an old and valued friend.*

This morning as I stood next to Carol's bed, she said in the most plaintive tones "Steve." At least my memory now some eighteen hours later tells me that was her tone. I can recall her expression, but I hesitate to label it lest my emotions intervene, but I will say it looked troubled. About what, of course, I have no idea. I believe I had just said my usual good morning and perhaps started, as is my wont, to chatter about the breakfast menu she would soon be offered.

Hearing my name, in whatever tone of voice, accompanied by whatever facial expression, in whatever circumstance, however everyday or not, whatever the context, always provokes a strong but ambivalent response.

On one level, I am pleased my name is still in her memory.

On another, I have no way of knowing whether she associates that name with me as I stand next to her.

I tried to clarify that point.

For her.

And for me.

"I'm right here," I say. "Steve is right here, as he always is."

She does not respond either verbally or with a change of her expression.

I go on chatting about the upcoming breakfast, the usual toast, breakfast sausage, juice, a fruit of some variety.

I suppose one day I will no longer hear her call my name.

I'm not going to dwell on that unpleasant eventuality.

Better to think about the weather. Will I be snow blowing tomorrow morning? I have no place I have to go this week-end, nor do I expect any visitors, so the weather is no great concern. I'll just listen to the wind and let it lull me into sleep.

Monday night. Carol asleep. The dog snoring.

Winter arrived over the weekend. I woke up to a snow-cov-ered driveway Sunday morning. Only a couple of inches so I didn't think it would be much of an impediment for me to deal with on my way to the store for Carol's muffin and my *Times*.

I was wrong. Underneath the thin layer of snow was a coat-ing of ice. I could not get past the end of the driveway where it grades up toward the road. At that point, the car just slid sideways. I tried a number of times giving myself more of a running start each time until I managed to sit on the edge of the road.

On the edge. Not on it.

It would be criminally stupid to back onto the road with-out stopping to make sure the way was clear. As it turned out, it wasn't. Cars coming one at a time from north and south. When finally the way was clear I tried to back onto the road. But lacking traction I went nowhere.

There was nothing to do but to put the car back in the garage, fire up the recently repaired snowblower and roll it out onto the driveway. It managed to take the snow off and just enough of the ice so that when next I reversed out of the driveway I could get up to the top of the driveway, pause, and then onto the road.

Which itself was covered in snow and ice. The four-and-a-half-mile drive to the store and back took at least twice as long as usual, as I kept my speed down to between 35 and 40.

Which almost seemed a bit too fast.

But I was dealing with conflicting pressures.

I did not want to leave Carol much longer than usual. But I also didn't want to risk an accident.

Now, I've been dealing with these roads in this kind of weather for sixteen winters. Ordinarily, I am confident and comfortable.

Not this time.

Because I could not permit myself to get stuck or worse. Carol was alone back in the house in bed. She cannot get out of bed to the phone, nor would she be able to use that device if it were within her grasp. I would not be able to call her, nor would she be able to summon help if she needed it.

As usual, I know I was not being rational in that my concern for Carol was exaggerated. Short of my being rendered unconscious, I would be able to summon help for her. Yet, I still found myself tense as I navigated the ups and downs and curves of the road. I was especially alert to the occasional oncoming car who might not be as careful or as experienced as I and so a head-on collision was not beyond possibility.

I pulled into the parking lot outside of the store, a little surprised that there were several other cars there, more than I would have expected on a bad weather day. But this is northern Michigan where people are not easily deterred from going to where they want to be. I bought Carol's muffin and the *Times*, exchanged pleasantries about the early winter with the clerk as I checked out and drove back still much more carefully than usual.

Not a bad thing.

And I was more than usually happy to get back home to ask Carol if she missed me.

I don't remember what she said.
It doesn't matter.

Tuesday night after a troubling day. Carol continues deal-
ing with accumulated phlegm, resulting in much coughing
and a gurgling sound as though she were drowning.

It was worse yesterday, much worse. At one point, I gave
her a little water, thinking, hoping, that it would somehow
do some good. What it accomplished was to cause her to
spew out a mixture of the water and the phlegm.

This was worrisome. I didn't know if something serious
was going on. I checked her blood oxygen, found it to be
98%, a very good reading, but I wanted more support, so I
called Chronic Care and spoke to a nurse. She asked me the
color of what was spewed. Clear, like water, I said. Any sign
of fever. No, I replied. And then, since this was someone I
had never spoken to before, questions about the history of
this problem, which I recounted to her.

By this time, Carol seemed to have settled down somewhat.
Less coughing, little gurgling.

The nurse said she would look into seeing what else could,
or should, be done. A little later, Chronic Care called to say
Clare, the nurse practitioner who usually sees Carol, wanted
to come tomorrow morning.

Pizza supper that evening with Ryan was almost as usual,
except Carol had little appetite and dozed off without eating
much.

The next morning at breakfast, she ate with better appetite. Still some sounds coming from her that I did not like.

Clare arrived, checked blood pressure, listened to her
lungs, announced they were clear, recommended I begin
again to give her Claritin, which I had stopped administer-
ing a while ago when the problem seemed to have mostly
disappeared. Clare said it would be good to suction out the
phlegm but that cannot be done in the home.

Then, she said, she wanted to have a serious talk.

About hospice, its advantages.

I listened and agreed to an evaluation.

But there is much more to be thought about and written about on that subject, so as it is beginning to get late, I'll tackle it next time.

The new normal for winter driving and perhaps a newer still version upcoming.

Hospice

Wednesday before Thanksgiving. Serious cold weather arriving perhaps driving temps into single digits.

Because I have been spending an inordinate amount of time working on my next column, I have a lot of ground to cover to catch up. I'll begin where I left off with Clare's suggestion that I consider signing up for hospice services.

The word "hospice" suggested end of life to me and that is why my initial reaction to Clare's mentioning it as a possibility for Carol was to want no part of it. When first I realized how serious Carol's illness was and at that time someone mentioned hospice for her my mind jumped to final arrangements. I even got in touch with a neighbor whose husband had recently died suddenly from a heart attack to talk with her about whom I should be talking to.

About final arrangements.

For Carol.

Because of the suggestion of hospice.

My original understanding, perhaps from media sources, was that hospice was a prelude to summoning the undertaker, a transition period when a dying person was made comfortable. At the time hospice was first suggested to me for Carol, I heard that to be eligible the individual had to be diagnosed as having some six months to live.

Thus, the thought that I should be thinking about arrangements.

My neighbor said she would put me in touch with the funeral director she had worked with. I said fine.

I didn't follow up, nor did she get back in touch. Perhaps she was waiting for me to take the initiative to proceed with preliminary discussions.

It was wise of her to wait on me because I was not ready so to do not only because of my obvious emotional resistance to the idea, but because despite Carol's cognitive issues she was quite obviously in good shape physically, a fact routinely confirmed by the medical professionals who on occasion saw her.

That is all background to Clare's bringing up the idea. She made it clear, however, that I was not to concern myself about that six-month mortality requirement. I now know that Medicare requires an assessment of eligibility in order to pay for the services hospice provides. Exactly what the basis for eligibility is remains a mystery to me, but it certainly does not involve a six-month prognosis. Once eligibility is established it is reviewed periodically.

In any event, having understood that my old understanding was wrong, and because Clare emphasized the services that would be available to us at no cost I agreed to at least explore the idea and Clare said she would set up an evaluation session to determine if Carol was, in fact, eligible.

Hanna, a nurse from Heartland Hospice, came the day after I called. She did the usual check of vitals, talked with Carol, I imagine to get an idea of cognitive functioning, saw that Carol's right arm was held stiffly to her side and resists having it moved, which makes dressing and undressing a bit of an issue, none of that coming as a surprise to me, of course.

Hanna had me trace, as best I could remember, the onset and progress of the disease. She inquired about what help I was now getting. She then announced that Carol was eligible for hospice, verified that I wanted to enroll her in it, which I did, as I now understood that hospice is a kind of Medicare-funded insurance program.

Got this difficult topic started. Will continue next time with the nuts and bolts.

Sunday night, the end of the four-day Thanksgiving weekend. Watched less television tonight because Poldark's season ended last week.

The most important service hospice offers is that Hanna will visit once a week. I am happy to have regular visits from a medical professional. I checked with Chronic Care, Clare's practice that has been supervising Carol's medical condition, to ask about coordination with hospice. It seems hospice is now in charge but that Chronic Care will check in every three months to verify that Carol remains eligible.

Although I do not now know, nor care particularly to find out what criteria made Carol eligible, I cannot imagine why she would lose that eligibility.

Some miracle improvement perhaps?

One should not try to find rational answers to the rules established by insurance companies, private or governmental. Just go with them.

Besides Hanna's regular visits, hospice will also send someone to the house whenever a situation warrants an immediate intervention, and that too is a comfort.

Hanna is a case manager, so all issues and services flow through her. Medicare, through hospice, pays for Carol's meds, and Hanna will need to stay on top of keeping me supplied since they are dispensed in a fifteen-day supply as opposed to the ninety-day supply my employer-based insurance provides. She will also put in orders for care items, such as hygienic items, or liquid thickener, that I have been buying but will now come to me cost free.

Also available from hospice are relief aides. Since all hospice services are paid for by Medicare, I could save considerable money by replacing my current relief aides with ones from hospice, but I declined to do so because I am well satisfied with the ones who have been providing that service for me for quite some time, a year or more, and I did not want to go through the process of working with new individuals.

I did contemplate replacing one aide to save that expense, but Hanna informed me that hospice aides only provide bed baths, which my current aides provide. They would not give me the block of free time I need.

Whether or not there was any truth that shaped my original foreboding about hospice for Carol, I am relieved and pleased to see that hospice has turned out to be so supportive without any of the negativity I had associated with it.

I had been handling this situation pretty much on my own. I now feel that although the disease will continue to do what it does, a support team now has my back and will be there to help me deal with whatever difficulties will inevitably arise.

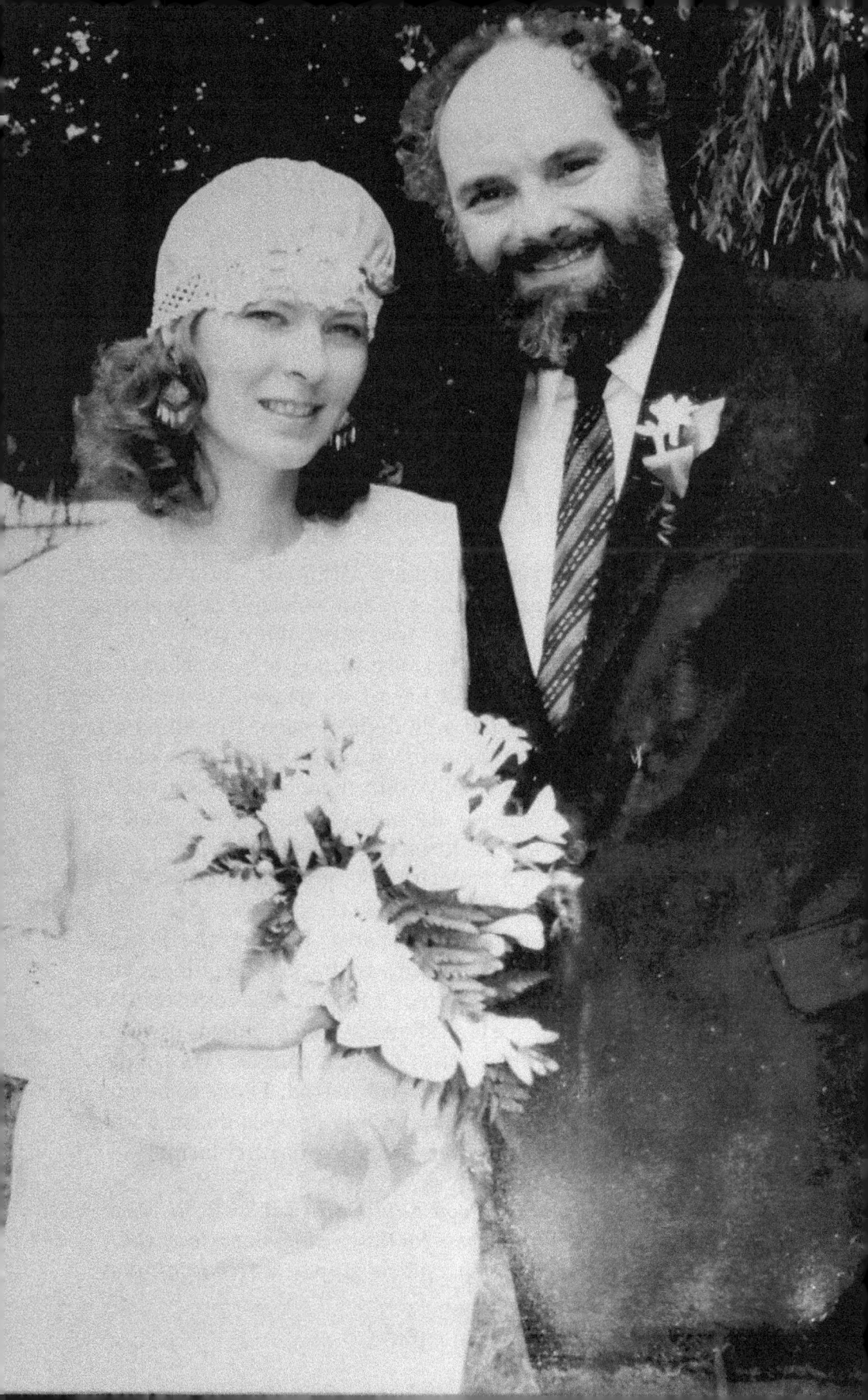

And She Said "Thank God"

Thanksgiving Day was quiet. I expected to get a dinner delivered from the Methodist Church community feast as that has happened in the past, as well as one from Brad and Amy who have thought of us on these occasions. We did receive both. We had the first on Thanksgiving, and the second on Saturday.

For some reason, this Thanksgiving I remembered one many years ago when Carol suggested we have lasagna. Which we did.

And shocked my two daughters although I doubt either now remembers. And I cannot recall whether they shared that meal or more likely I just told them about it.

Nor am I sure why we made this culinary choice other than to suggest that perhaps neither of us wanted to deal with a turkey and all the usual side dishes. Also, thumbing our noses at conventional behavior was probably part of the motivation, as we used to have our chocolate mousse before the main course when we ate out at our favorite spot on Montague Street near the Promenade in Brooklyn.

In any event Carol's appetite was good for both of this year's very typical dinners.

Her appetite has improved because Hanna, the hospice nurse, ordered atropine eye drops to dry up the phlegm that has been accumulating in Carol's throat. As counterintuitive as it is to use an eye medicine for this problem, it works. I apply a couple of drops onto Carol's tongue twice a day, and the phlegm issue is largely eliminated. I have to be careful to make sure that the drying out process doesn't work too well and begin to interfere with regular urination.

Monday night after a good day. Carol ate well all three meals, laughed from time to time, and slept less than usual. Ryan joined us for a pizza supper, which reminded

me how much I miss Papa Nick's New York pizza. Men-
tioned that to Carol and she seemed to agree that the loss
was incalculable.

The other morning as we were getting ready for the day, Carol said, in the plaintive tones she sometimes uses in articulating this word, "Steve," uttered with a look on her face that indicated something was bothering her, or perhaps scaring her. As I was standing right next to her bed, I took her hand, and said, "I am right here, Steve is right here," and gave her hand a little squeeze for emphasis.

"Thank God," she replied, articulating those two words quite clearly.

I've been down this road so many times before, it is both a little tiresome to repeat the obvious question but necessary at the same time.

Did she connect the physical me with the Steve she was summoning? That her response "Thank God" seemed so heartfelt only adds to the significance of the question. It is good, of course, that the Steve in her head, whether connected to the Steve holding her hand or not, is somebody she still feels bound to, someone whom she can call for when troubled.

But here is the recurrent dilemma. Perhaps it is not such a good thing after all because it reinforces the idea that we are still suspended between the then and now heading toward a future at which point the then might disappear, at least for her.

It will always stay with me.

I don't want to leave it, and I cling to every instance when it reasserts itself, cling to it while acknowledging that doing so is, in the long-range view, futile.

A start. Much more to explore with no hope of finding a
comfortable resting place.

Sunday night. A cold wind blowing outside. Carol asleep
under the new blanket I ordered online for her on the

advice of Hanna who thought the afghan I was using was not warm enough because of its loose weave. Carol and I have always had very different thermostats.

Have not been writing in my journal that much this past week, not because of any problems, but rather the absence of difficulties providing me with time that I have decided to devote to my writing career. I am aggressively marketing two unsold novels and writing my columns as ideas occur to me. And now, once again it is late, and so I will just try to pick up where I left off, hoping to spend a good writing session on it.

The "it" was provoked by Carol's response to my insistence that Steve was standing right next to her bed holding her hand to which she replied, quite clearly, "Thank God," raising the continuing dilemma of how to deal with such emotionally fraught moments.

Of course, one part of me is delighted for a couple of reasons. First, the answer in its clarity illustrates a good level of cognitive functioning. As new as I am to dementia, I have no measuring stick in terms of movement up and down along a scale of cognition other than the everyday observation that there will be good days and not so good days.

In that regard, recently I have not seen much fluctuation. It is true enough that Carol does not often articulate clearly enough for words to be apparent, but occasionally she does. And perhaps more to the point, she seems these days more responsive to direct questions that require a yes/no response, such as "Are you hungry?" which sometimes elicits a strongly positive response. In addition, she is laughing more at particular things I say, sometimes comments directed at the dog over whom I occasionally trip, or just old dog that she is, decides to plop down right in the path of the wheelchair. And, finally, in this brief survey of her cognition, I am fairly well convinced that she listens intently to the music I have playing throughout the day. I have asked her from time to time whether she is listening, or whether she is enjoying the music and she usually responds in the affirmative. I have also seen her moving a foot in time with the rhythm she hears.

So from that perspective, her "Thank God" response fits that pattern.

But it also raises that other bothersome issue, namely, whether or not she connects my name with my body. There is no way to get a good read on that. I push sometimes, but do not get a definitive answer to that question.

Which in some ways is quite important.

Because it underscores the tension in my situation between knowing I have to let go of my sense of Carol as she was and my not wanting so to do.

What occurs to me as a way to explore this tension is to focus on my moving between our upstairs bedroom and the couch on which I now sleep.

That will be for next time.

The Persistent Past

Wednesday night after a busy day, starting with my going to town for regular blood work while neighbor Wendy stayed with Carol. While I was out, the podiatrist visited to cut Carol's toenails, and then after I returned Hanna arrived for her weekly visit.

Carol is still in her chair, and I will need to move her to the bed in a little while, so I will just get something started.

I sleep on the couch near Carol's bed. Every morning I go upstairs to shower and change my clothes for the day. I have been doing this for quite some time ever since Carol was no longer able to climb the stairs and we were both sleeping on the couch before I ordered the hospital bed for her.

As routine as this trip upstairs has become, my sensibilities are still shocked, like a splash of cold water in my face, as the reality of the fact that never again will we share that bedroom, yet it remains exactly as it was before. Carol's robe, which she no longer wears, is still on the hook on the door to the peculiar little closet that has been carved out of a corner of the room. Next to her dresser, neatly sitting on the floor, are her winter boots, and next to the bed, her slippers, pink like the robe for which it was bought as part of a set.

I could go on and catalogue other items from our previous lives together in that room, but the point simply is that the room looks exactly as it used to.

Before.

The bathroom the same. I have not removed her towel from the towel rack, or the economy size load of her Q-tips from the shared closet that served as our medicine chest, or the glass bottles, sitting on a shelf across from the sink, blown by her former boyfriend, relics of a failed relationship that we rarely discussed.

The entire upstairs is like a museum. To remove any object would be, it seems to me, a desecration.

A start. The well is dry for now.

Tuesday night after a day that began with some good news. An editor at a university press whom I queried a couple of days ago about Carol's story collection wrote to say she would take a look at it. These days even getting one foot in the door is difficult. I have no doubt the collection is well worth publishing, and hope this editor agrees.

Besides acting as Carol's agent, I've been spending more time pursuing my own writing career, sending out queries for my unpublished work and also writing columns for my new once a month—soon to be twice a month—responsibility. This is healthy for me. I loved teaching, got satisfaction as an administrator, but at the core I saw myself as a writer who did other things to pay the bills.

In my last writing session I was riffing on my two bedrooms: the one Carol and I used to share, and the makeshift sleeping arrangement now in the living room. Going into our former marital bedroom for fresh clothes draws me back to what is lost. That motion is constant like the tide on a beach working its way up the sand before withdrawing again, the back and forth repeated endlessly.

That might work for the tide, but it's not a comfortable way to live. I need to feel something that represents movement away from that dip into the past upstairs and the return to the present downstairs every day. The same back and forth holds true for the times I work in my office next door to our bedroom where my new desktop PC beckons although I do most of my writing and other computer work on my laptop while sitting in my armchair across from Carol's bed.

My life as a writer provides that forward thrust away from the untenable past. True, it is an element from that past but continuing it now is like walking away from that beach, perhaps after spending time in the ocean waves. You can't stay in those waves. You either let them drown you, or you break away from them.

Focusing on writing, both producing and marketing, is a way for me to free myself from the clutches of the pull between the present and the very intense connection to the past.

I don't at all regret or resent assuming my caregiving responsibilities and intend willingly to continue them as long as my strength permits me.

But I do not want to lose myself in them.

Sunday night approaching midnight. In the absence of Masterpiece *for my usual television viewing I watched a football game. Having played some football myself, and having been a lifelong fan, I can watch any game that is competitive enough to hold my interest.*

Yesterday evening as we ate supper, the radio, as usual, was tuned to the Interlochen station. As is inevitable this time of year, that station's programming was immersed in the holiday season. However, the program that came on as we ate offered an interesting variation by presenting an hour of Hanukkah-themed music, even though that holiday had already come and gone. What made hearing that music yesterday at dinner a little odder was the fact that during the afternoon I had retrieved our miniature artificial Christmas tree.

Our piano sits at the intersection of our dining room and living room. The radio had been on one side of the instrument closest to the living room. I moved it to the side of the piano farthest away from the living room so I could place the tree on its spot. I plugged in the lights and after lunch wheeled Carol over to the tree so she could see it, and she responded with an appreciative smile.

So, last night at supper, the radio playing Hanukkah-themed klezmer music was on one side of the piano while the little Christmas tree with its blue lights was on the other.

A perplexing, almost jarring juxtaposition of the two traditions to which neither of us adhered with much intensity.

And a not unpleasant intrusion of the past, an idea, perhaps, worth exploring in more significant ways looking toward the future.

Christmas

Friday night. Carol in her chair, the dog sleeping on the floor. Snow falling as befits the official start of winter. Even though I spent some money to get my old snowblower repaired and ready, I decided to contract with the landscaping company that does my fall cleanup to take care of snow removal. I just don't want to have to deal with that issue. If this deal gets too costly, I still have a reliable snowblower.

This is the start of an extended period of isolation, longer than my usual weekend break, because this coming Tuesday is Christmas Day, and although I could pay extra to have my relief aide come, if she were willing, I chose instead to switch her to Wednesday. I usually do food shopping on Tuesdays, but stores won't be open. Nor will the library where I sometimes go to work. So, I just moved everything to Wednesday.

Not a happy prospect. But Ryan is coming for his usual dinner Monday night, and rather than plan on our take-out choices I bought a petite roast. I haven't cooked one in quite a while, and this seemed like the right time.

Otherwise I guess I'll spend more time writing and reading. And that is not a bad thing.

Saturday night a few minutes after midnight. Just finished sitting with Carol, holding her hand, as she drifted off to sleep. As I settled into my chair, the dog decided her day was also over and strolled to her bed.

The first day of the long stretch between relief aide visits leading up to and past Christmas. A little snow on the ground, just enough to please those who believe the holiday must be white but not enough to pose a problem.

I guess kind of the best of both worlds although I could do without both.

The day went by easily and fast because it was filled with digital contact with my daughters. I hadn't heard from Danielle for a while and so I sent her a text to which she responded, and we caught up with each other messaging back and forth. I sent her a picture of the 1998 ornament on the little artificial tree, and she responded that she remembered making it. As much as I would like to see her, it seems a visit home for her is still a ways off.

A piece of music from Interlochen Public Radio provided the impetus for me to get in touch with Kerri and Tracy, as well as including Danielle in the ensuing messaging. The station played a track of a klezmer band doing its version of The Little Drummer Boy.

I was perplexed. I couldn't figure out whether I was more irritated or more amused by the extraordinary marriage of Jewish musical style performing a tune celebrating the birth of Christ. Klezmer music is upbeat and happy, played at weddings and other celebratory events. To hear it employed for this Christmas song was just weird. There is no other word.

So weird that I thought I'd share it with my daughters, two raised in Jewish households, and one in the Carol and Steve combo. Religion was not prominent in either of those households.

Of course, I would have loved to be able to talk to Carol about this musical experience, but she had slept through it and in any case would have only been able to offer a small response, a smile, or a frown, or perhaps a word or two.

But whatever it would have been I would have been happy to receive it. I'm pretty sure she would have been ambiguously amused. Klezmer music is hard to resist, and she wouldn't have approached this performance from my more complicated perspective.

As it turns out, and as I learned later, Tracy was preoccupied and so did not respond to my message. Kerri, on the other hand, did and we discussed it through a number of messages. We first checked to determine if the klezmer band is in fact a Jewish band. It is. We agreed the track was weird, not just strange, or different, but requiring a stronger descriptor. Weird will do.

To share the music, I found a YouTube version by the same band. That version of course has images, and the images, in cartoon figures, emphasized the religious message of the birth of Christ, which is not as prominent in the song as heard but not seen.

Adding those images sealed the deal for Kerri and me, as we agreed that whatever the band's motive in producing this track was, the result was disrespectful to both traditions.

And yet, at least for me, that judgment is offered with a lingering smile.

Christmas Eve after a good dinner featuring the roast with Ryan. Carol asleep in her chair, the dog as usual stretched out on the floor.

I had trouble finding music to listen to today, even on the classical stations. I have no objection to Christmas-themed music but what was offered today just wasn't that interesting. Ditto popular music with somewhat less tolerance because, well it's popular music made primarily to cash in on the holiday and is just otherwise not that good. When I heard the fourth or fifth version of Rudolph, that time by Dean Martin, I had had enough and put on a CD of Pavarotti doing serious holiday music. I could listen to him sing the alphabet song.

Carol seemed indifferent to the music until she heard Pavarotti singing *Ave Maria*, and then she perked up.

During the afternoon an unexpected visit from Jane and daughter Marissa bearing gifts, followed by a long overdue catch-up conversation particularly with Marissa who will be finishing college in a year.

That socialization followed a weekend of long-distance parenting with my daughters.

With Kerri, as described above, messaging about the

klezmer band playing Christmas music, with Tracy a phone call later about various issues that she was dealing with, for which I served as a sounding board and one-person support system, with Danielle the next day, an extended conversation concerning a life decision she faces, for which I was not so much as a sounding board but rather a source of fatherly advice.

Three daughters, three different interactions, all of them filling my usually isolated weekend with the reach of long-distance interactions.

These interactions turned my head toward the future, reminding me of the ongoing parenting roles available to me, valuable in themselves, but more so as a mechanism to help me break my brooding chain to the lost past with Carol.

And just as important as breaking that chain is the strengthening of my resolution to continue my caregiving role with Carol by putting it into a larger context, one that extends beyond the possible limits of those caregiving responsibilities.

Just trying to keep my legs underneath me and my head on straight as I travel along this unknown road.

Toward the Light

Thursday night. Christmas has come and gone. Carol and dog asleep. I have just finished cutting about five hundred words off a story so that it almost slides under the word limit of the market to which I want to submit it. I figure I'm close enough, and there is no more fat to trim.

As always, I enjoyed the pruning process, which is where the necessary craft in writing is usefully applied, where the writer must remove himself or herself from the product being produced and attempt to see it as readers will. That is a hard-learned skill the application of which is a source of satisfaction.

We are getting through this holiday decently well. My relief aide schedule had to be rearranged because both Christmas and New Year's Day fall on Tuesday. Nothing much will be open on either day, not stores, or the library where I sometimes work. We switched my Tuesday aide to Wednesday after Christmas and to the following Monday before New Year's Day. Today, I had no one come because of a vacation issue with my Thursday aide. I could have perhaps agreed to a replacement who had never been here before, but that just didn't seem worth doing.

Tomorrow, I'll have my usual lunch with my guys.

The holiday season will soon be in the rearview mirror. We are on the other side of the winter solstice so even though we are just entering the long northern Michigan winter, snow on the ground and more to come, I prefer to think that we have turned the corner and are heading toward the light. It may be distant, but each day when the sun hangs in the sky a little longer is a positive.

I try to convince myself that this meteorological fact will somehow have some parallel in my life. I cannot, literally, move out of the darkness of Carol's disease. No increased sunlight or metaphorical light can accomplish that magical feat for me. But I've never been satisfied with the status quo, whatever that might have been. I always believe, whether with reason or not, that things will somehow get better.

And there are signs that may be the case now. In several ways, I am experiencing more people interactions, both with Carol's family, with my daughters, albeit long distance, and with a variety of respondents to my newspaper columns, those mostly of the digital variety. It seems as long as I keep making myself available one way or another, people will respond.

And that is a very good thing.

Friday night, dog snoring on the floor to say all in her world is just fine.

Sent an email to my lunch companions containing a link to a review of *The Penguin Book of Hell* in the *New York Review of Books*. I thought they would be interested in that subject as we had touched upon it this afternoon as tangential to our discussion of morality. Our lunchtime conversations do move between the largely inconsequential to the serious. But that is not why I mention this email. I saw that it went out under Carol's name because the periodical's account has been in her name for some years from the time she renewed it.

Renewed it for me.

She never read that periodical whereas I've been reading it most of my adult life. Just one more of so many reminders of the care and respect we extended to each other. I recall subscribing to *Scientific American*, which I don't read, for her. And so it went.

And now I'll do what I can for as long as I can for her.

Sunday night after midnight. Spent the day between care-giving responsibilities and watching a lot of football.

Although as I have recalled, Carol never evinced much

interest in football, she had begun to show some interest in fast-moving games like hockey or soccer. But what she watched with most interest was basketball, the game she played herself, remembering as she reminded me more than once that she had been captain of her team in school. If we found a women's basketball game to watch, she would settle back and enjoy it.

She would watch baseball with me, and root hard for the Detroit Tigers. I imagine her interest in this sport was at least in part associated with her father who was a fan, and who was, so Carol told me, named by his father after the famous old-time pitcher Walter Johnson.

For those who enjoy competition, and Carol in her way, certainly did, sports is an acceptable outlet. Carol's ambitions as a writer was just another expression of her innate competitiveness.

I, too, confess that I am more than a little competitive. I do like to win.

But I can say with honesty we never competed with each other. As I write this, it occurs to me that statement includes any form of competition, be it a game of checkers or Scrabble. It could be that Carol just did not enjoy those kinds of games although I certainly do.

As sugar sweet as it may sound to say, the answer might be that we wanted each other to do well in whatever we were doing. In games with winners, there have to be losers. And just perhaps we did not want to see the other person lose. As corny as that sounds, and although I have never thought about this question literally until this moment with my fingers banging down the keys of my laptop, it may well be true.

There are different kinds of light, those provided by sun or moon, those captured in metaphors of hope emerging from darkness, and those that memory shines on those whose lives are so inextricably intertwined with our own.

At the center of all of these, for me, is Carol.

New Year's Eve

New Year's Eve, about twenty minutes until 2019 arrives. I am quite sure that at 12:01 the world is going to be pretty much the same.

I am, as I was last year, listening to WQXR streaming from New York, and as it was last year the station is offering Beethoven's 9th. I will keep it on so I can hear the wonderful "Ode to Joy." As I did last year. Some things remain the same. Ah, here comes the Ode. Will it end at the stroke of midnight?

Because of the holiday tomorrow my Tuesday aide came today, but a little later than usual as the first consequential snowstorm had arrived and was finding its voice. Snow or no snow, it was my grocery shopping day. Driving into town, around town, and then back required patience and care especially on the Peninsula where visibility was limited and the roads slippery.

Still, I did as I had planned. I did my three-stop food shopping and then picked up Chinese takeout for supper with Ryan. Carol ate with good appetite, and Ryan and I chatted until it was time for him to go home about eight thirty. It took him some time to get through the snow on the driveway and out onto the road. I thought, at one point, I would have to go out and push when he was stuck, but he managed to rock himself out.

After dinner, I thought I'd watch a little television only to find that the satellite signal was interrupted. I trudged out to the dish in the backyard and scraped ice and snow off of it. That restored the signal, but I soon found there was nothing I cared to watch.

I am trying to get into the New Year's spirit and not doing a very good job of it. The whole thing, of course, is absolutely arbitrary. Yes, the earth orbits the sun in a year, but where we choose to mark the beginning point, and therefore the ending point, is just picking a place on a circle and placing your finger on it. Until the middle of the eighteenth century, the new year started in March at about the time of the vernal equinox. That certainly makes as much sense as the first of January. As that day arrived, I am pleased to report that Beethoven's Ode sailed right on through midnight. For another four minutes or so. Not much. But it is the principle. We do not have to be in thrall to the clock although I confess myself usually guilty of too much time awareness.

So, I am nitpicking instead of celebrating. Or coming up with resolutions. Let's try the latter.

I resolve to be less time conscious. To let life breathe on its own.

Nothing could be more important as I continue dealing with Carol's condition. I'm looking for patience and forbearance.

Some measure of both for me, and a bit more to spread around among those who have not found a way to be a part of this situation.

Tuesday night, reaching the end of the first day of the new year, which greeted me with six to eight inches of freshly fallen snow coating the ground and anything on it. However, to my immense relief I saw that my driveway had been cleared while I was still asleep. Later in the morning Rocco came by on his riding snowblower and neatened up the first job. I thanked him and alerted him to my contract with the landscaping company. He said he would just come by when he had the time to see if more needed to be done.

Aside from my brief conversation with Rocco I spoke to no one else today. Even the phone was silent, either because it was a holiday or more likely because the push to sign people up for Medicare Advantage programs has ended for now. I posted a picture of the snow on Instagram and Facebook to invite responses and received several. I guess I need to feel connected when nobody is scheduled to come by.

Just took it easy for the day, attending to necessary chores and giving myself a good nap when Carol was dozing, as she usually does, in the late afternoon. I read one long review of a biography of Thomas Cromwell, a key player in the turbulent years of Henry VIII. Besides my usual interest in people and events historical, Cromwell is featured in the two novels by Hilary Mantel covering this period. They are superb historical novels, and I await the forthcoming third in the series. The reviewer of the biography declared that Mantel made educated guesses to fill in what the historical record did not offer. As a writer of historical fiction myself, I understand that the story must move along. It can't just stop where the record is mute. Nor can you let the facts get in the way of that movement. Mantel is masterful.

I am reminded that Carol, too, had a strong interest in history in two particular directions: local and feminist. In terms of the former she departed somewhat from the usual focus hereabout on the settlers and subsequent farming families. Her interest extended to the Native American populations who appear regularly in her stories. As for the latter, she was a quiet but determined feminist as titles on her bookshelves make abundantly clear and her female characters are strongly drawn.

Tonight, after supper I spent some time watching television, more than I usually do. There really wasn't any news on, which ordinarily I would have checked in on, so instead I tuned in to a little college football. After catching parts of a couple of games, which did not hold my attention, and with no news being broadcast, Carol asleep, and not feeling like reading, preferring to veg out in front of the television, and reminded by an ad arriving in my email that as a library card holder I was also registered with Hoopla, I decided to see what it could offer for my entertainment, and found the film version of Philip Roth's *The Human Stain*, which

331

I read some years ago. The film featured some good actors, including Anthony Hopkins, Nicole Kidman, Ed Harris, and Gary Sinise, so I tuned in to it. I didn't remember the novel well enough to judge how good a job the film adaptation was, but the movie was, as you would expect with that cast, well-acted. After a while, though, I was reminded that the plot device Roth used to drive his story strained credibility. Still, the film did its job of providing a couple of hours of decent entertainment.

Neither Carol nor the dog were up for a discussion of the film, so I joined them in sleep.

And so 2019 began.

A Most Difficult Decision

Friday afternoon in the community library. As I pulled into the parking lot I saw several dozen, or perhaps more, children going up and down the large hill at the side of the lot. Those going down were doing so on their bellies. No sleds. I'm guessing they were enjoying recess time from their classes.

Yesterday morning, I received a text message that Carol's uncle of whom she was very fond had died. I've been thinking about that message in two very different ways.

The first way was the wording of the message, which stated that the uncle was completely healed. I was, reasonably I think, at first a bit confused. Healed from what? Injury? Sickness? The question popped into my mind. The next sentence answered that question by announcing that the viewing would be at such and such time, with the service the next day.

So I understood. I will return to the cause of that initial confusion and what that confusion leads to for me.

The second, and more significant, response to that news was a different question, namely, should I tell Carol? Maybe the answer either way seems obvious, but it was not, and still to a certain extent, is not so clear. I've been anticipating facing this situation in terms of Carol's mother who has been for several years in a skilled nursing facility. She is, I believe, 94. About the same age as the uncle, who as far as I know had been living by himself although always with his daughter, Carol's first cousin, nearby.

The uncle's death, then, arrives within the context of the preparatory thinking I have already been doing concerning Carol's mother. The decision I have made after wrestling with the question since I received that message, and in part based on a couple of more professional recommendations, will likely guide me in deciding what to do when Carol's mother's turn arrives.

The first professional recommendation came in a purely coincidental conversation with Hanna, our hospice nurse, late Wednesday before the text message concerning Carol's uncle arrived the next morning at seven o'clock. I do not recall why I raised the subject with Hanna, but I shared with her my question as to how I should handle Carol's mother's death. I do believe my opening concern was securing relief coverage that would enable me to attend the funeral, which would be announced with little precise forewarning. Hanna assured me that hospice would patch together some kind of coverage.

Having settled that concern, I moved on to the deeper more difficult issue. Should I at that time tell Carol that her mother had died? Hanna answered the question by reflecting her own experience that suggested that the only time she had observed a problem with informing a dementia patient of the death of a loved one was when that patient, lacking memory, but still capable of verbal expression, would repeatedly ask after the person who had died, and not remembering that she had been informed that the person had died would have to be told each time that the individual was no longer available.

In Carol's case her verbal expression is severely limited, and I cannot measure her memory loss with precision. She may no longer know who I am, but she seems perfectly comfortable with my caring for her. Not too long ago, but still not recently, she would occasionally call out for her mother, and I would assure her that she was being well cared for where she was in the facility, and that comforted her.

So Hanna's informed response did not help me much as my unanswerable question concerns whether there's a place in Carol's inaccessible long-term memory for her mother.

Is her mother still in her mind?

I don't know. I suspect not, but I cannot be sure.

If she is, wouldn't it be the right thing to do to tell her when her mother dies?

Maybe yes, maybe no.

My rational self tells me that no is the better answer. What point would there be to giving Carol any sorrow at this juncture in her life?

My emotional self, however, feels that I would be doing her an injustice if I didn't tell her something so vital as the death of her parent.

The balance was shifted to the negative today, albeit perhaps only for now, by the answer I got to the question from Tonda, the very experienced aide. Tonda simply declared that in her view Carol would not understand what I was talking about should I tell Carol her mother had died.

For all her experience, though, I am not sure Tonda is right because there continue to be instances where although Carol lacks the ability to articulate her words, she does definitely seem to be processing what she hears and responding to it facially or with a laugh, or with the one or two words she can still say. In that latter regard, a week or two ago, she uttered a complete sentence, "You can't do that," apparently to some thought in her mind.

In less fraught situations, I deal with this question when Carol, as she is doing now, receives birthday wishes, or a note from some friend or acquaintance, which still occurs, coming from people either unaware of, or the degree of, Carol's dementia. In those cases, I have no problem passing on the greeting to Carol and cannot say with certainty as I sit here typing whether the names of these individuals register. It doesn't seem to matter. These correspondences do not arrive with any emotional baggage.

But the ones concerning her mother, and by her extension her uncle, are certainly in a very different category, one for which my decision, at least as I see it, is consequential.

So without clear guidelines based on discernible evidence, the question remained. My head argued with my emotions, and my head prevailed in that it could see no good outcome to telling Carol her uncle had died. If he still resides in her memory and resurfaces into her conscious mind at some point, I decided, let it not be spoiled by the fact that he is no longer a part of her life.

Whether my decision concerning Carol's uncle will set the pattern for her mother or not, I cannot at this point know. Likely it will, because Carol shared a deep and abiding bond with this man, not equivalent to the one with her mother, but not very far short of it.

In any event, I have arranged for Wendy, our very accommodating neighbor, to stay with Carol while I attend the viewing.

Returning to the phrasing of the news from Carol's cousin, that metaphorical view of life as an illness from which at death one is cured immediately took root in my brain as something worth writing about. And, no doubt, that root will grow into a column, which is already forming in my head, an exploration of the different ways in which writers over the centuries have presented attitudes toward death.

But for the present, it is enough to say that writing about this difficult decision has brought it into a focus, has placed it out on the table where I can poke it, turn it over, and make up my mind.

And that is the best I can do.

Snow

Late Sunday night. More snow expected overnight and into tomorrow.

About six inches greeted me this morning. What didn't greet me was the service I had contracted with to keep my driveway clear. I wanted to make my usual Sunday morning trip to the market.

I eyed the driveway calculating whether I would be able to drive over the snow and up onto the road. I had already put on my snow boots to trudge across the road to pick up the local paper. That walk back and forth over and through snow drifts argued against trying to back my car out onto the road. That now seemed like a really bad idea with the prospect of my getting stuck at the edge of the road where the snowplows deposit their loads. I started to walk back into the house. After all, I could serve Carol her regular breakfast featuring toast instead of the Sunday muffin.

And I could read the *Times* online as I do when the paper is not available at the store. And it was about five degrees and windy, so getting back into the relatively warm house seemed like a good idea.

But not good enough.

A combination of my dedication to routine and irrational urge to get Carol her muffin even though, if I thought about it, I am sure she would be indifferent to the breakfast menu *sans* muffin, these factors pushed me to get my car out. I also recalled that I had spent a fair amount of money getting my old snowblower in shape before I had decided to save myself the stress and strain of snow removal and contracted with the service that had failed me this morning.

I went back into the house to don my ski mask, extra heavy double gloves containing one pair within another, flipped up my hood to cover my hat, walked into the garage, propped open the door with my splitting wedge to clear my egress behind the snowblower and onto the driveway.

I primed the snowblower, set the choke, maneuvered my clumsily clad fingers onto the pull cord handle and yanked.

Nothing.

Yanked again. And again.

Still nothing.

Right after it had been serviced, the snowblower had started at the first yank.

Not today.

I can be stubborn when an idea has rooted itself into my brain. I remembered that I had a spray that encouraged noncooperative engines to start. I located the can, aimed it at the carburetor intake, sprayed. Then checked the choke and throttle control, just to be sure, grabbed the pull cord handle, and yanked. With a spark coming from the intake, the engine roared into life.

It took me about fifteen or twenty minutes to clear the driveway. At one point, I almost walked out onto the road in a whirl of blowing snow that hid an oncoming car. Fortunately, I saw it in time.

By this time, my hands, in spite of my gloves, were achingly cold, as was I, and tired as well from all the effort. I came back into the house, sat down to rest and wait until my fingers stopped aching.

I told Carol that I was now off to the store.

I returned a little later.

With a muffin and the paper.

Carol had her usual Sunday morning breakfast, and about that I felt very good. Admittedly an irrational feeling, but still enough to lift my mood as I sat down to read the paper.

Tuesday late. The wind is howling outside, and snow is coating the windows. We are in the midst of an on-again, off-again snowstorm that is supposed to continue into Thursday.

I managed to get into town to do my shopping. Driving in I encountered a couple of near whiteouts from blowing snow, and the roads were icy. Driving in these conditions always makes me uneasy with the thought of Carol lying helpless in her bed. I know my concern is exaggerated, that sooner rather than later she would be taken care of should I be disabled.

But knowing that does not free me from the concern.

My plan today was to get my shopping done fast enough to leave me time to go to the florist we had been patronizing since moving here seventeen years ago and pick up a flower arrangement for Carol's birthday tomorrow. I checked with Lexie, today's aide, and she said she could stay a little while longer if necessary.

My timing worked out even better than I expected so I finished my last stop at the grocery store on Eighth Street and drove east the few blocks to the florist.

Only to find out, and then to recall, that it had closed. Not for the season, but closed, as in out of business. That florist had been in business for seventy-two years and picked now to quit. Actually, not now, as I was reminded when I checked online: it had announced its closing last July, but I had not remembered.

I still wanted flowers for Carol, knowing, once again, my emotions were triumphing over my reason since the latter told me that it was an open question as to how tuned in Carol would be to her birthday. In the best of times, she was largely indifferent to the calendar although she was careful to keep a list of family birthdays that she could consult. Her indifference was to time in general. For birthdays, or appointments, she required some form of external prompt, such as a datebook.

Now, of course, she is even less aware of what day it is. Still it is her birthday. I will read to her the few birthday cards that have arrived from those who apparently share my conviction that we need to honor the day whether or not she can be made aware of it. With that in mind, once I got home and had with Lexie's help unpacked the groceries, I looked up florists in town, found a couple, chose one that had the best review and called up. I had an unexpectedly pleasant conversation with the person who took my call. She asked if I were from New York. I confessed I was born and raised in Brooklyn. She was pleased. She said she thought so, being herself from New Jersey, and so we agreed we were both fish seriously out of the water.

I ordered an assortment that would be colorful but left the details to her. My knowledge of ornamental flowers does not extend much past roses. They will be delivered tomorrow. I will show them to Carol and read her cards to her. I am aware that I am insisting on doing all of this even knowing that if I let the day pass by without notice of its significance, Carol would be every bit the same as she is.

But I would be unhappy, remorseful, an obligation unfulfilled, one that belongs to the Carol that was.

On this one day I am perfectly fine with that.

Major and Minor

Monday night after a couple of days of warming that pro-
vided a respite from the polar vortex that drove tempera-
tures to below zero with highs topping out in the single
digits. It was small comfort to know that a wide swath
of the country was experiencing the same and worse. In
such circumstances, the old saw that misery loves com-
pany rings hollow. Misery yes. Loving the company. Not
so much.

As if to somehow emphasize the point, the cold air hitting
the back of my neck after breezing through the window air
conditioner reminds me that the cold has returned.

I hear Carol restless in her sleep as she usually is. Between
me and her on the wood stove sit the flowers that the bad
weather, whiteouts, and icy roads caused to be delivered a
day late.

Not surprisingly, her birthday came and went with little
notice. The weather was so bad that not only were the flowers not delivered but Hanna did not come out for her weekly
visit.

However, Jane did stop by late in the afternoon when I was
napping. I did not hear her if she rang the bell or called out.
She messaged me later to say she had left a card and gift for
both of us on the bench in the entryway. The gift turned out
to be a package of mini brownies and the card featured a historical photo of the Peninsula's volunteer fire department
in 1945. Each member in the picture was identified and I
recognized some of the old family names. Thoughtful gifts,
both, and I regret I was not awake to receive them properly.
Jane did say that the dog had done her best to welcome her.

I brought the flowers to Carol. She seemed not to react
to them. I read Jane's card, as I had the others that had
arrived. I detected some level of recognition.

It is clear that all of my preparation for her birthday, like so many things, such as insisting I get a muffin for her on Sunday, are much more for me than for her.

That is not surprising.

The noisy little electric heater just kicked on. I have my earbuds on tuned to jazz from KNKX, Seattle. The buzz from the heater almost drowns out the music.

I got a bit of good news and not so good news. The good news came yesterday when I saw a notice that the new issue of *Rosebud* magazine containing my Holocaust-themed short story has just been published. I am in good company with this fine little literary mag based in Wisconsin as this issue includes a conversation between Allen Ginsberg and William Burroughs. I have no idea how that conversation has surfaced so many years after the death of both of these counterculture icons. I'll have to find out when my contributor copies arrive. When they do, I'll order a few more copies to send out.

And I'll announce this latest publication to the world. Whether the world will be duly impressed is another question.

But every publication reinforces my commitment to my writing career. In this instance, this publication encouraged me to send out two queries, one for each of my unpublished novels.

The not so good news came today in a telephone call from my dermatologist's office to inform me that the growth removed from my scalp last Thursday was precancerous. My doctor is sure she got all of it and will have me back to take a look in six months, so clearly there is no urgency.

Still I would have preferred to have heard that the growth was innocuous.

It wasn't, and naturally enough raises my concern not only for myself but for Carol. In that regard I tell myself I've done all I can to prepare for the possibility of my predeceasing her. That is good, but not something I want to dwell on.

I think I'll end on that note for tonight.

Saturday night, quite late.

Thursday I went to town to at long last deliver to Munson Hospital the final wishes document I finished preparing a while ago. I suspect I was delaying doing this task because on some deep level it required me to think about end of life matters. Of course, I know I should do that planning, as unpleasant as it is, and so I dutifully went through the forms, got the appropriate signatures for patient advocates, indicated what I want done with my dead body, and how I want to be comforted before breathing my last, all of which is well to document now, but clearly pertains to a situation I have shoved into a closet in my mind to be taken out only when the urge to put the matter to rest motivates me to open the door to it.

I also have a couple of loose ends from setting up my trust that I need to attend to. Nothing that consequential, but again I find little motivation to take care of them. Which is not like me. Generally, I do not like things hanging over my head that I know must be attended to.

It is likely that my present unanticipated situation is providing me with a somewhat different frame of reference for these kinds of decisions. It will take some work to unravel that idea.

I can start that unraveling by setting out an incident seemingly of much less significance than end of life planning. When I came home from my lunch yesterday, I intended to retrieve my mail before settling back into the house. I pulled into the driveway, hit the button to open the garage door, eased the car in, got out and walked back onto the driveway, my eye across the road toward the mailbox.

Which wasn't there.

A snowplow had knocked it off. The post stood naked. When I got to it, several feet away in the snow, I saw the box still attached to the crosspiece that had been bolted to the post.

End of life planning on one day, and a mailbox problem the next. I'll take a look at each in turn.

If Carol were well, it is likely that I would not yet have filled out the papers I just delivered to Munson Hospital, let alone set up a trust. Perhaps at my age, my previous indifference to these matters was irresponsible. Carol and I did have wills, and I probably thought that was sufficient.

I remember that years ago we had investigated purchasing insurance that would pay for assisted living or nursing home care should either of us reach that stage. But the cost for such insurance, as I recall, was exorbitant at our then ages, so we dropped the idea, settling for each of us having a will. Other than that, we assumed we would take care of each other.

I'm doing my best to hold up my end of that supposition.

It is, however, a more complicated story when I think about how I reacted to the mailbox being knocked off. Naturally, I was irritated. But more or less than I would have been before Carol fell ill?

It seems to me, I should be considerably less concerned about my mailbox on the day after I filed my last wishes and walked into the house where I would take over Carol's care from the relief aide. If I imagine one of those ancient scales, the kind with two shallow bowls suspended from a fixed arm that pivots to one side or the other depending upon which bowl has the greater weight, in such a scale the side containing my emotional attitude toward contemplating the end of my life would, I imagine, lean down much harder than the other side containing my irritation at having to repair a mailbox in the dead of winter when beneath the snow the ground was frozen solid making replacement impossible until the spring thaw.

While yet alive, I can avail myself of work-arounds to the mailbox issue if repair is not possible. Life would go on albeit, perhaps, with some inconvenience. However, I don't recall any place on the forms I filed at Munson concerning the receipt of posthumous mail.

So why do the petty concerns bother me as much as they would if I weren't acting as Carol's caregiver, and in that context making sure she would be taken care of?

I think the answer is that part of me remains consistent with the man I was, and that man never reacted with equanimity to certain relatively minor assaults on his sense of how the world should be.

Such as there being in that world a mailbox remaining upright and available to receive mail.

That I still value that kind of mundane element in my environment, is as important to me as my admittedly much more important responsibilities. In fact, that retention of who I was enables me to be what I have to be now.

Her Book

Monday night. Jazz from KNKX in my earbuds. The dog slurping water from her dish. Carol quietly and peacefully asleep, which is both welcome and a bit unusual.

Spent the day in the house with the electric heater trying to provide a little warmth against the cold aftermath of the blizzard that roared through last night and into the morning. Looking out of the kitchen window while getting breakfast ready, I was pleased to see my driveway already cleared. I had no plans to go anywhere during the day, but it is always good to know I can get out if I need to.

I received several congratulatory responses to both my column published yesterday as well as my announcement concerning my short story publication. It's hard to quantify such occurrences, but I would say there was a definite uptick, including hearing from friends and family I had not been in contact with in some time.

All well and good.

But in spite of that attention directed toward my writing, or perhaps because of it, I spent some time trying to make good on my intention to find a publisher for Carol's story collection. A Google search brought up a list of possibilities broken down into three categories: big house, academic, and independent.

I don't think it useful to spend time checking out big houses since I am reasonably sure they would require to be approached through an agent, which at this point I do not have. I will take a look and hope to be pleasantly surprised.

I scanned the independents and found three whose names are familiar to me. A couple that looked promising will open for submissions on March 1. Among those supported by universities, a number seem to want work to be submitted to a contest. Interestingly, I never liked that approach for my own work, but Carol, on the other hand, not only did but won recognition in doing so. I guess I should pursue that approach both because it is hard to avoid and maybe some of Carol's good vibrations will work again. These contests all charge a reading fee. I just don't like the idea of paying somebody to read my work. I suppose part of me, driven by my not inconsiderable ego, believes it is their privilege to be given the opportunity to read what I have written. The same holds for Carol's excellent work.

I do recognize these publishers, even with university support, could use the money to offset costs, and perhaps as well need to limit the number of submissions to those serious enough to pay a few bucks. I don't recall Carol paying such fees years back, but maybe she did.

In short, very few writers and/or publishers make much money from short story collections. The fees, from that perspective, make a certain amount of sense.

Friday is March 1, and I will send out at least one submission.

Tuesday night after midnight. The forecast is for three to five more inches of snow arriving by late tomorrow afternoon.

My recollection is that Wednesday's weather has been bad more often than not. Fortunately, I don't have to go anywhere on Wednesdays although Hanna makes her weekly nurse visit on that day. This week, though, Hanna is in Hawaii, and I do not know if someone is scheduled to come out in her stead. I suppose I'll find out in the morning.

At the butcher shop today, I bought a pork tenderloin and a small roast. Both anticipate a dinner with Ryan. Last night, I cooked up a pork tenderloin with his assistance. I had intended to make it for Carol and me but saw that it was big enough for the three of us.

Which it was. Just barely.

Carol seemed to enjoy the meal, as did Ryan and I. That success encouraged me to plan on a repeat, and as long as

I was in that frame of mind, I bought the roast for another time.

I never claimed to enjoy cooking, but the take-out possibilities here are not particularly appetizing. The Chinese takeout is closed on Mondays for the winter, and there are just so many mediocre pizzas I feel like eating.

So, I'll do a little cooking for our Monday night dinners.

Shopping day tomorrow. I should get some sleep.

Wednesday night, quite cold, but no wind or falling snow. Portable electric heater doing its best to provide a little warmth.

Spent way too much time watching the Michael Cohen hearing today, but I am a news junkie. Cleansed my viewing palate a bit tonight by watching a good hockey game even though my team, the Rangers, lost.

This morning, I stood by Carol's bed and pulled up the blinds and looked out at a light snow shower. Nothing too serious but still most unwelcome.

"Carol," I said, "It's fucking snowing again."

She laughed. Which raises the question as to what amused her.

Perhaps it was the expletive.

Or maybe just her northern Michigan heritage.

The first is more interesting and requires a bit of context.

I'll begin by saying I am bilingual in this way: I can do the Brooklyn street argot of my youth or that of the English professor, complete with doctorate, of my adult life, and pretty much anything in between, depending upon my mood and circumstance. In the Brooklyn of my youth, becoming comfortable cursing was a rite of passage. I can't explain why that was so in my circle. In truth, I never heard my parents or other adults in the neighborhood utter even a mild profanity. They were probably aware that profanity was associated with the lower classes with whom they did not want to be identified. As for us, their children, maybe that class sensitivity was the reason we cursed, to differentiate ourselves from our staid, striving parents. After all, these were what the poet Robert Lowell called "the tranquilized Fifties" that soon gave way to the raucous sixties. In the middle of that tranquilized decade, Allen Ginsburg published his profanity laced "Howl," which is a literary version of what we were doing on street corners at night, offering a middle finger reprimand to all that social climbing niceness.

Be that as it may, profanity became a natural part of my linguistic toolbox, available for humor or anger. I recall our daughter saying she learned curse words from me when we were stuck in an interminable traffic jam on the Merritt Parkway approaching New York from Connecticut.

Coming from a very different background, Carol did not curse much, if at all. In searching my memory as I sit here writing, I cannot bring up a specific memory of her using profanity although I believe she did on rare occasions. I just can't be sure. What is true is that I am keenly aware, after seventeen years living on Old Mission Peninsula, that if folks here curse they must do it outside of my hearing.

Carol never expressed any unhappiness with my every once in a while cursing. Maybe she just thought that was the Brooklyn part of me coming out. She had loved living in Brooklyn, the energy and the expressiveness of its people as contrasted to the reserve of those she had grown up among. She told me many times that she enjoyed and respected that expressiveness.

So maybe that was what she was responding to this morning. I hadn't used the f-word in anger although perhaps a little bit in frustration. It was just a modifier, an intensifier. To have just said, "Carol, it's snowing again" would have been inadequate. It wasn't just snowing yet again. It was fucking snowing again.

There is a difference. And I suspect that is what Carol was responding to. I want that to be the case. I think it shows that from time to time, perhaps more often than I am aware, she is in the moment with me.

And I treasure those moments, not so much for her sake.

But for mine. And getting her book published, if I can manage it, holding it in my hand, will in a much larger way serve as a physical manifestation of all the moments I want to remember of our lives together.

Just Letting It Be

Sunday night a little after midnight. The dog is snoring loudly, an uneven accompaniment to "After Hours" played by Gillespie and the two Sonnys, Stitt and Rollins, in my earbuds from Pandora.

It's been a quiet weekend with a little more snow but nothing serious. The Times *hadn't arrived at the store when I came for Carol's muffin, so I read parts of the paper online. I had done the Sunday puzzle online last night. Watched hockey and baseball this afternoon and the season-ending episode of* Victoria *tonight.*

Carol just laughed in her sleep. She does that from time to time although perhaps less often than she had been doing. I don't know whether to attach any significance to the change in frequency.

More importantly, it opens the door, once again, to speculation as to what is going on in her mind to which she no longer can give voice. But that there is some cognitive or memory activity seems beyond doubt, and trying to penetrate the mystery of that something demands my attention even though I know that I will never be able to peek behind the screen of her disease to discover what prompts that occasional laugh. A joke? An incongruity? A physical stimulation caused by her movement in the bed?

I have not heard her say my name in a long time, yet it seems clear to me that on some level she knows me. Perhaps not as her husband. Maybe as her caregiver. Maybe not even anything as specific as that.

When Tonda left Friday afternoon, after commenting that she had had a good day with Carol, she said something like, "I'll leave you now with your beautiful wife."

Of course, whether or not Carol still knows that she has a

husband, I think of her, even in her reduced state, as very much my wife.

Which leads me to a thought I have been having lately, namely, my reaction when people, in all good conscience, compliment me for being a good husband, for taking such good care of my wife.

I am doing the best I can to make Carol's quality of life as good as possible. For example, I picked up on Tonda's suggestion, after all this time, to raise the blind next to the hospital bed, which I had kept down to keep out the draft, and then have Carol lie on her right side, so she could look out of the window at the huge lilacs on that side of the house.

She must have loved the outdoors, Tonda had opined.

Indeed, she did.

And perhaps still does.

The constant question.

How much of the then Carol persists in the now Carol? I've gotten used to her new normal, grafted it, in a sense, on my memory of her as she had been. I am holding on to that composite of the once was and now is Carol.

When I am complimented for my good care of Carol, I want to say, "But yes, I am doing this for me as much, and perhaps more, than for her. It is possible that were Carol in a facility her care would be as good, maybe even better, than what I can offer. At least, it would be professional. I am taking care of her in our house because I cannot imagine, at this point, being without her physical presence in my life."

But I don't say anything like that because anyone who has not experienced what I am living through couldn't, despite his or her best efforts, understand. So, I just accept the compliment and say, "We're doing the best we can."

Not, I'm doing the best I can. But we are. Because I insist there is still a we.

And I also tell myself, with some justice, I can give Carol what no nurse or other medical professional can and that is a bridge to whatever memory, however faint, she retains of me and our life together.

That is no small thing.

But I still haven't touched on the other side of the coin. Which is I am standing on the other end of that bridge reaching toward her, so I can bring myself to her.

In deep waters. Will pause.

Tuesday night. The dog, after rousing herself to walk into the kitchen to slurp a drink of water from her dish, has settled into her bed. The electric heater, set to automatic, has just turned itself on filling the room with its noisy hum. Carol is sleeping peacefully on her side.

That is the important fact with which to start this writing session.

Carol usually sleeps, rather restlessly, on her back, from which position she manages to still get her feet jammed between the mattress and the bumper, or sometimes even to throw her leg over the top of the rail. In that position as well, she usually breathes noisily through her mouth.

But now, her breathing is quiet, and she is mostly still.

About an hour ago, she fell asleep with my arm around her and my hand in hers. We were lying together on her bed in the spoon position. Reaching this point evolved over several stages. At first when it was time for her to go to sleep, I leaned over the bed and held her hand. I noticed that this contact seemed to settle her into a sleeping mode, and so I would wait until her eyes began to close. Then, I would say good night, release my hand and fix the blanket around her.

But standing in that position, sort of leaning toward her, was difficult to sustain for the length of time it took for her to reach sleep. I began to sit on the edge of the bed. But that, too, was a bit awkward as the back of my thighs pressed onto the top of the lowered side rail. I began to shift my weight toward her with my arm across her chest to reach her hand. Again, I was not happy with that arrangement. I did not want my body weight to come down on her and it was a bit of a strain to prevent that from happening.

Thus, the spoon position, in which both of us would be comfortable, I would still be holding her hand, and the same relaxing into sleep process occurred.

None of this would have mattered if I were going to just wish her good night, and then go about my business, just like I always used to do. But now I enjoy watching her relax into sleep. For that moment, all is well in our little world.

When she feels my presence, she relaxes. I stay with her like that for a while until her breathing gets regular as she drifts into sleep. I cannot explain why she reacts this way. I imagine she feels safe. Perhaps a shard of memory from our past sleeping together in the same bed rises from some distant corner. In a way, her reaction in this situation is an amplified version of what has always seemed to happen when I take her hand. On those occasions, as well, I noticed a calming effect, and sometimes what appeared to be a reciprocal pressure, a bit of squeeze around my fingers. I thought, then, and do now still believe, that such a response might well be more neurological than emotional.

But maybe not.

I simply cannot know.

I have decided that I don't have to. What is more important is how I feel about these occurrences, particularly when I have my arm around her and hear her regular sleep breathing.

At those times, I am holding on to a memory. Or more precisely, I am recalling that memory. And, I too, for those moments, feel at peace. I know nothing about our situation has changed. She will not miraculously get better and be the person she was. That is not going to happen.

Yet, in those moments, without conversation, it is as though we have agreed to just live in that moment and not ruin it by burdening it with analysis or expectations or regret or hope or anything else.

Just let it be what it is.

And that is more than good enough.

For it establishes a way for me to deal with the perplexing and frustrating task of living with what remains of the woman who has been so important to me every day for almost forty years from the beginning of my middle age to where I now sit in my senior years with the prospect, perhaps, of outliving her, and so face my own end alone.

And so with due apologies to Paul McCartney, without asking any help from Mother Mary, with no attempt to sing the line on key, but with a bit of Brooklyn emphasis I insist that I will just damn well let it be.

Of Then, Now, and the Future

In the community library on Thursday afternoon. With my computer on my lap, I have just finished an edit of the post that I will publish Saturday morning. My neighbor, a senior citizen of my vintage, sitting to my left is doing some kind of low-tech work using an actual pen hovering above a piece of paper while he studies the page of a magazine.

A nostalgic and refreshing sight.

This morning for the first time in months, Carol said my name. She might have been a little stressed as I got her ready for the day. For whatever reason, she looked in my direction and clearly articulated "Steve." Later in the day, but much less clearly, she seemed to say my name again.

A short, but meaningful messenger from the past, announcing that it is not quite dead. Some form of me still resides in her brain, available to her under certain conditions, whatever they might be.

And to whomever, specifically, that form is directed, the me sitting next to her, or the remembered me.

I don't, at this point, try to pin that distinction down, nor do I really care.

What I do care about, as I have written about before, is that there is some form of we still alive and, if not well, at least hanging on.

Rather than ponder the imponderable, there are practical matters to deal with. In that regard, the first thing I did when I arrived at the library today was to draft a letter to the insurance company that holds a life policy on Carol. We took it out years ago, calling it her funeral money. And I suppose that is what it still is.

We thought then that my retirement funds would certainly cover putting me in the ground, or in the cremation furnace, but there was no similar pot of money for Carol. Of course, the money that would take care of me, could just as well serve for her. But, if my memory is right, Carol in her usual way wanted this matter to be taken care of in her own way. In her own name.

Thus, the policy.

My task today was to make sure that the money would be available to whoever would be responsible for Carol's end of life arrangements, should I predecease her. I am now the beneficiary of that policy, and so it seems a good idea to put a next beneficiary in the event of my already being gone.

The letter I drafted to the insurance company asked that our daughter be added as the next beneficiary. No doubt, there will be more paperwork, but this is a start. When I get home, I'll print up the letter and an envelope in which to mail it.

One more thing about to be taken care of.

This chore leads into the thoughts I have been having about the possibility that the predeceasing might go the other way, for in spite of Carol's being ten years younger than I, her disease might eliminate that advantage.

She might die before me.

That is a really unpleasant thought.

Sunday night. Woke up to more snow, wet and heavy. Driveway not cleared; road not plowed. I decided discretion was the better part of valor, fought off the tug of entrenched habit and routine, and chose not to drive down to the store for Carol's muffin and the possibility of picking up the Times. *The road just looked dangerous with several inches of wet, heavy snow. Although there were tire tracks, so some vehicle had come by at some point, there was no sign of any traffic now as I waited for ten or fifteen minutes before making up my mind to stay home. This winter does not seem to understand that we are a week away from St. Patrick's Day, followed by the first day of spring.*

Had to set the clocks ahead last night, and because I got up at the usual time, I lost an hour's sleep. That, plus the snow, started the day off on the wrong foot. But Carol had a good breakfast, I did the Sunday *Times* puzzle online and read a bit of the paper, watched a little baseball, served Carol pork chops with applesauce for dinner, which she enjoyed, and finished the day viewing a very nice fundraiser special on PBS showing an ancient but very well-preserved Tony Bennett working with the much younger and vibrant Canadian jazz singer Diana Krall in the process of making an album. Their music was wonderful, but even better was seeing how they worked out their back and forth handling of the lyrics, and how the piano player leading a trio including bass and drums added his view of how the song should be presented in terms of the intro and pacing.

After the show ended and it was time for Carol to head toward sleep, as has become a habit, I lay spoon-wise in the bed with her with my arm around her until her eyes closed and breathing became regular. She is sleeping now but restlessly for some reason. I can only guess her mind is active, exploring, or remembering, or inventing. For example, I've noticed a new indicator of some kind of cognitive activity. When she was listening to a piece of music, her left hand seemed to be mimicking the movements of playing the piano. It did not look spasmodic; rather the movement was more controlled, going from left to right and her fingers, so it appeared, doing a little up and down action. I can't be sure, but that's how it looked.

I do guard against reading innocent signs into something more significant, so I offer these observations to myself while admonishing myself not to take them too seriously.

And yet, the impression came to mind with an immediacy that argues for my having seen something of note. I'll keep an eye out for a repetition.

All of this, the going to sleep routine, the meals, the close observation tell me, as if I needed to be reminded, how much a part of my life Carol remains. It's the reason that after more than a year, approaching two years now, I think, at the expense of my back I still sleep on the couch so that I can hear her breathe. There is really no practical reason for me to do that. She is perfectly safe in the hospital bed.

But the thought of being on a different floor overnight just does not work for me.

I am sneaking up on the topic I thought I would be working on tonight, namely, my thoughts concerning the possibility that Carol might predecease me.

I'll try to attack it next time.

Out of time for now. My neighbor still hard at work. I'll leave him to it and head home.

Like A Body Blow

Tuesday afternoon of a lovely spring day. I notice in my journal a remark from about a week ago: Just saw a blue jay land on the table on our deck amidst the still-falling snowflakes, and shake its feathers as though to say what the fuck is going on?

The blue jay if it is still around would be happy today, sunshine decently warm, temperature about forty, snow melting.

I, on the other hand, for reasons I will set out when I get back some energy, find this lovely weather in complete opposition to my mood, not because I don't, as the blue jays no doubt do, luxuriate in the return of spring, but because that return of spring and all it suggests is particularly difficult for me to contemplate after the events of the last six or seven days.

I am writing when I am usually resting after coming back from my weekly shopping excursion, and I am way too tired to continue. Will pick it up perhaps later tonight. But what I have to say must out. And soon.

Tuesday night. Dog snoring, Carol sleeping. I've turned off the late baseball game I was watching. It is time to uncap what has been brewing in my head.

What started last Wednesday morning is what makes this glorious springlike day hit me like a body blow. Spring is a time when we see life waking up again, particularly after the harsh winter we have just endured. So while that is what, I expect, most folks are feeling, that feeling in me is crushed under the weight of an approaching dark shadow.

At breakfast last Wednesday, Carol experienced a choking episode, apparently on a piece of breakfast sausage, the same kind of breakfast sausage she has been eating for years before the onset of her disease and all the way through it. The night before, she had eaten the usual frozen lasagna that I serve on shopping days. The night before that, she had eaten pork chops with me.

So although I have been aware for a very long time that swallowing issues are absolutely predictable as her disease progresses, and although there had been minor signs of that difficulty, I was not prepared for the chain of events triggered by that episode last Wednesday.

That afternoon, she developed a fever of something over 101. I called hospice, and a prescription for an antibiotic was phoned in to the pharmacy in town. Ryan came and stayed with Carol while I fetched the antibiotic, which I administered over the next couple of days. I also noticed even more phlegm accumulating in her throat, some of which I was able to scoop out.

I canceled my relief aide on Thursday and stayed home to monitor Carol's condition. The fever came down somewhat, and she seemed to be recovering. The cause of the fever was determined to be that bit of sausage, getting into her lung, which I learned is highly susceptible to infection. On Friday, she seemed on the mend, so I joined my friend John for lunch. I had been serving her easily swallowed yogurt since the incident. Because my stock of yogurt containers was running low, I asked John to drive into town with me after we ate so I could buy some more of the coconut-based variety that Carol needs because of her lactose intolerance. He came along, and on the way back he was in the car when Hanna called, and I discussed with her what foods I could safely add to Carol's diet and when I should do so. She recommended continued caution because of the danger of a repeat choking incident. When she came for a visit, she reiterated that warning.

By Saturday, I was feeling uneasy, and felt I wanted confirmation that we were over the hump of the infection and that her lungs were clear. I called hospice, expecting to ask for a visit from a medical professional on Monday. Hanna had told me that there would be a nurse on duty over the weekend, but to my pleasant surprise I learned that meant the nurse would come out to our house.

He did. He confirmed that Carol's temperature was normal and that he detected no continuing problem with her lungs. We discussed food possibilities, such as bread, crust removed, with peanut butter for protein. Greek yogurt because of its high protein quality. We were looking for easily swallowed but nourishing foods. I jotted down a tentative menu.

The weather was warming up, and my spirits were rising with it.

But there was a warning sign. I admit that I was anxious to see Carol on a more normal diet, so I called Chip, the covering nurse on Sunday to check with him about what I was thinking of serving for dinner—elbow pasta with pesto sauce, a dish Carol always liked, as she was particularly fond of pesto. Long ago, she made her own. He thought it would be alright but recommended that I cut the pasta pieces into smaller chunks. I did, but Carol did not seem interested in them. I switched to chocolate yogurt, and she ate most of one container decently well. She had little interest in the protein drink I also served her. At that point, I was not too concerned about her mixed dinner appetite since it was not unusual for her to have little enthusiasm for either lunch or dinner, and I supposed this was an occasion when her dinner appetite was limited. I had certainly observed that kind of thing before.

I was not prepared, therefore, for what followed.

On Sunday, I had picked up some Greek yogurt. I served that yogurt to Carol on Monday morning, but she did not swallow it, nor did she have much interest in the protein drink. She almost always has an appetite for breakfast, so this was concerning.

Hanna came in the late afternoon just before Ryan arrived

for our usual supper. Her prognosis after examining Carol was devastating. First, she found a sore on the roof of Carol's mouth, which she attributed to acid from food being stuck there rather than being swallowed. Then she observed a choking fit when Carol was served some yogurt.

She said that it was time to consider switching my thinking about food from providing it because it was nourishing to withholding it because of the danger it presented of a fatal choking episode. She also, in answer to my question, indicated that the phlegm I was observing in Carol's mouth was the result of swallowing difficulties and not the sole cause of those difficulties. Not being able to swallow efficiently prevents dementia patients from getting the phlegm down their throats as healthy people can do. Limiting it, as we had been attempting, is helpful, but not a definitive answer.

Wednesday evening. Carol in her chair having eaten some of her supper. It's a little early for me to write, but I want to keep this section going with the hope of perhaps picking it up later after Carol is asleep.

I understood Hanna's concern, but I confess I was not ready to concede that we had reached the point where withholding food to initiate the slide into death had arrived. After Hanna left on Monday, and after Ryan and I had our dinners, I swabbed Carol's mouth as I had been instructed to do.

To my pleasant surprise, she was clearly swallowing the water in the sponge-like head of the swab. Swallowing it without difficulty. Ryan confirmed what I was seeing.

The next day, by coincidence Clare from Chronic Care, the supervising practice responsible for Carol's being in hospice, was scheduled to come by to continue certifying her eligibility. Hanna arranged to be there at the same time. I deliberately did not attempt to feed anything to Carol before they came. I wanted them to witness what I hoped they would see: Carol still able to swallow.

I had pureed some bananas, which Carol had been able to eat on Sunday morning.

With Hanna and Clare watching, Carol ate the pureed bananas. They went down without much apparent difficulty. The two medical professionals agreed to hit the pause button on moving toward withholding further attempts to provide food.

Just a pause button.

I know that. And also know there is no way to predict how long the pause will continue.

Hanna was here today and insisted on that point, and I didn't need the insistence. This disease has been a very effective, if harsh, tutor for me. And I have been a stubborn, resistant, but ultimately accepting student of its hideous machinations.

Will stop here to catch my breath.

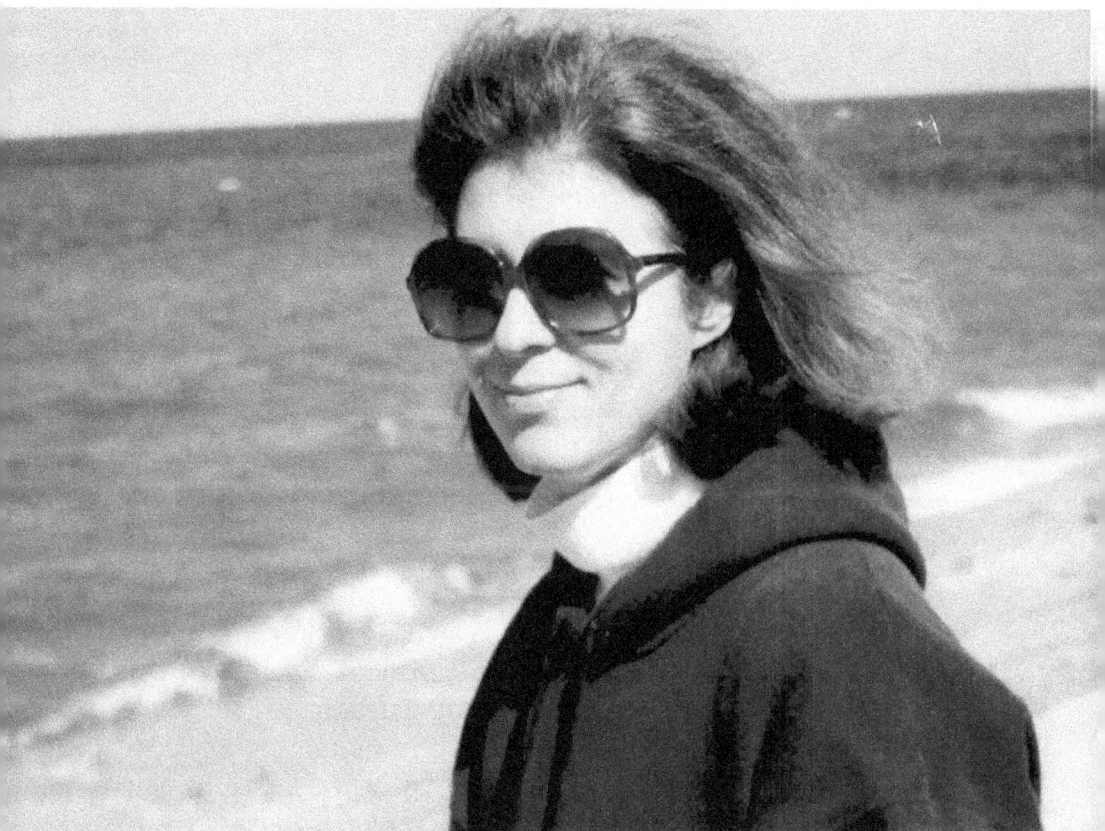

Fin

Thursday afternoon in the community library during my respite period. I had contemplated staying home up in my office to either write or begin the odious chore of getting my tax material in order for my appointment next Thursday with my new tax preparer. Because I am really not in the mood to confront that necessary chore today, and because I am pulled to continue writing my way through this extraordinarily difficult period, and because getting out of the house is always a way to recharge my batteries a bit, I am here. The tax material will still be waiting for my attention.

Hanna has been coming almost daily, but she is skipping today. Yesterday, Nic, the hospice social worker, visited. I was glad he did. I was going to call him to invite him out but when I came home from shopping Tuesday afternoon, I found a message from him on my landline phone.

I had been thinking about talking to him as a follow-up not just to all that had been happening over the past week, but specifically as a result of a suggestion that my brother-in-law Ward had made. He called me as I was on my way into town to do my shopping and we wound up speaking for close to half an hour, much of it while I was parked in front of my first stop at Burritt's meat market. What stood out in that conversation besides Ward's very welcome supportive comments was a particular, very practical suggestion: I should now make sure whom I would call when I would be facing Carol's lifeless body. I'm expressing the idea more bluntly than Ward did, but that is what we were talking about. You would not want, he had said, at that stressful, emotionally wrought time, to have to figure out how to deal with the practical necessities, specifically the person or agency to call. And beyond that to at least have some idea of how I wanted to handle the final arrangements.

I had thought, if I had thought about that unthinkable yet inevitable, moment at all, that I would call hospice. I believe my Tuesday aide had suggested that idea when I told her about Ward's conversation. That seems and seemed reasonable but would not have sufficed because at that point I would still have to figure out who should be contacted to perform the necessary end of life service of collecting the body. Contacting hospice would, in effect, just transfer that decision to it. It would be well for me to have researched possibilities and, if possible, to have made a decision. I surely could still call hospice, who could then take over the necessary calls, including the one to the funeral parlor service I had chosen.

Ward's suggestion turned out to be prescient.

From that point in my conversation with Nic, and being absolutely without any experience organizing a funeral, and never really having given that process any thought, I asked him to provide me some basic information.

Which he did, including, at my request, some estimates of cost, as well as possible services that would be offered. He asked if I would like to have more specific information. I said yes, and he agreed to call several places of good reputation. I had told him that my preference, as far as my thinking had gone, had been abundantly clear that I wanted something simple, small, and private. I also intended within those boundaries to respect Carol's family's wishes as well as I could.

This morning, I received an email from Nic reporting on his research into the several companies he had mentioned. I am now prepared to make a decision.

A decision that is crushingly difficult to contemplate. I have acquired retrospective respect for all those grievers who organized the funerals I in the past have so mindlessly attended.

I have been keeping Carol's siblings and my daughters

informed. I asked the siblings to communicate these sad tidings to the extended family. I am aware that Danielle, our daughter, now intent on leaving her current job as well as the state of Minnesota, is in the process of long-distance interviewing for a new position in Pennsylvania. She said she would find a way, whether or not she gets the new job, to spend some time with me and her mother.

I also, in the context of pursuing my intention of getting Carol's story collection published, contacted friends at Mission Point Press, and informed them of the turn Carol's condition had taken.

I might send separate emails to particularly close life friends, and perhaps a few writers who knew us as fellow practitioners.

As devastating as all of this has been, as emotionally overwhelming as it no doubt has been, and will continue to be, I find a little relief in brushing off my ancient administrative tools to work my way through this uncharted territory.

Doing that, and finding the time, energy, and inclination, to keep my writing career going by producing columns, keeping this journal and from it creating blog posts, and occasionally, still, marketing my work, all of that is necessary to keep my equilibrium.

Time to leave the library.

Friday afternoon, eight days after the above. I am in my office at my desktop and will summarize those intense eight days.

On the previous Friday, Carol's swallowing difficulties had increased. I stopped trying to feed her nourishment. Hanna and I talked about transferring Carol to Munson Hospital Hospice on Monday. I agreed with Hanna's suggestion to hire a private duty caregiver, who arrived in the early evening. She was willing to stay around the clock until Monday morning although she was not sure we had that much time.

She would keep Carol comfortable, her mouth moistened, her position changed, and any pain deadened by a steady dose of morphine.

I told Danielle that now was the time for her to come for what looked like a last visit. I also kept daughters Tracy and Kerri in New York informed. Danielle set out from Minnesota and arrived Saturday evening, a little after Allison, the private duty caregiver had arrived and had taken over responsibilities.

On Sunday evening, after what were now regular visits from the hospice nurse, Danielle and I went out for dinner at the familiar restaurant down the road across from the market after waiting for the hospice grief coordinator who was scheduled to come. She was delayed, and so I informed hospice to tell her we were going out and she could visit tomorrow.

As we were about finishing our meal, my phone rang. It was Kristi, the grief coordinator. I began to apologize for postponing her visit until tomorrow.

As soon as I got those words out, she said, "Carol just died."

She asked if I wanted to stay at the restaurant while they took care of things. I said we would be home in a few minutes. Once there, when the workers from the funeral home came, I talked with them as to the best way out of the house, and then sat in the green room until they were gone.

I did not want to witness the removal itself. I had said my good-bye with a kiss on Carol's still warm forehead, looked for as long as I could tolerate, only a few seconds, at her still very pretty face.

Danielle stayed through Monday, and then got in her car to travel back to Minnesota. Tracy flew in from New York and arrived not long after Danielle left. She provided immense comfort over the next few days as I, along with Ward and Jane, met with the funeral director and worked on composing the obituary. When I wasn't writing, Tracy was there to talk to or just as important to be there when we were both working, she on the work she had taken with her, and I on the obituary. When the funeral director called, I put him on speakerphone and asked Tracy to listen to what he said with her attorney's head, so I got things right. I was not thinking all that clearly.

Ward and Jane helped me disassemble the hospital bed and move the pieces into the garage. I did not want to see it.

I went about informing friends and relatives.

Arrangements that had to be made have been made. There will be a graveside service. With the help of the family, I have written the obituary, and made plans for a memorial reading of Carol's stories.

This hideous journey is over.

Epilogue

At ten thirty at night, I sit in the green room watching a March Madness basketball game without much interest because one team is getting thumped and the outcome is not in doubt. I think about finding something else to watch because I am an hour or two short of my usual bedtime.

But the clock turns my attention to the hospital bed in the next room. Isn't it time, in a few minutes, to settle Carol for the night? To make sure she is clean and comfortable? To climb into the bed with her lying on her side and throw my arm around her, take her hand, feel, perhaps a responsive squeeze from her, stay there with her until her breathing announces her sliding into sleep?

But she is not there.

The hospital bed is disassembled and in the garage, waiting to be disposed of some way, along with all the other medical equipment associated with her illness.

I realize that for the past two years or so I have been living a fiction of my own creation that I was still living with the Carol I had loved so deeply for so long, a fiction fed by occasional real or imagined responses that encouraged me to continue talking to her, to tell when I was going out to get the newspaper or the mail or upstairs to shower or that we were going to move into the kitchen for breakfast or to the dining room table for dinner, what we would be eating at either of those meals, to sit with her while first I fed her meal to her, her own hands useless, watching her swallow and drink, finish meals with her meds in applesauce, and on certain days plan how to use my respite time whether shopping or having lunch with my buddies or working in the library, and then back home again to pick up the same routine from morning to when the clock reached just about eleven at night after which I would work on my laptop for some time and then settle down myself onto the couch a couple of feet from her bed, where I could hear her restless movements and her breathing.

But not now.

That book is closed.

I must somehow start a new one.

Later, upstairs in my office.

I reach over to my desk on which sits the ancient, manual perpetual calendar reading August 12, the day Carol could no longer climb the stairs up to our bedroom and her long decline began.

I turn the device's wheels to today's date.

And so I begin.

About the Author

Born and raised in the Flatbush section of Brooklyn, Stephen Lewis holds a doctorate in Puritan American Literature from New York University, and he is Professor of English Emeritus at Suffolk Community College, on Long Island, New York. He now lives in a restored farmhouse on Old Mission Peninsula in northern lower Michigan.

His first novel, *The Monkey Rope* was published in 1990 followed by *And Baby Makes None* (1991) two mysteries set in Brooklyn and published by Walker & Company. Mysteries of Colonial Times, were written for Berkley, and drew upon his expertise as a scholar of New England Puritanism. *Murder On Old Mission*, put out in 2005 by Arbutus Press, was a finalist in the historical fiction category of *ForeWord Magazine's* book of the year awards. His mystery novel, *Stone Cold Dead*, was submitted by Arbutus to the 2007 Edgars. Mission Point Press in 2017 reissued *Murder On Old Mission* and published its sequel *Murder Undone*.

He has published six college textbooks and now writes a regular column for the *Traverse City Record Eagle*. Most recently, he has arranged the posthumous publication of *The Wolfkeeper*, his wife's short story collection.

As his wife's caregiver during her losing battle with early onset dementia, he wrote a blog that became this book.

NOVELS:

1990 *The Monkey Rope*. Walker & Company. A mystery.

1991 *And Baby Makes None*. Walker & Company.
A mystery.

1999 *The Dumb Shall Sing*. Berkley. A historical mystery.

2000 *The Blind in Darkness*. Berkley. A historical
mystery.

2001 *The Sea Hath Spoken*. Berkley. A historical mystery.

2005 *Murder On Old Mission*. Arbutus Press A literary
historical novel.

2007 *Stone Cold Dead*, Arbutus Press, 2007. A mystery.

2013 *A Suspicion of Witchcraft*, Belgrave House,

2017 *Murder Undone*, Mission Point Press, sequel to
Murder on Old Mission
Reissue of *Murder On Old Mission*, Mission Point
Press

TEXTBOOKS:

1972 (with Edward Eriksson) *Focus on the Written Word*,
Norvec, a composition rhetoric.

1974 (with R. David Cox) *The Student Critic*, Winthrop,
an introduction to writing about literature.

1983 (with Cecile Forte) *Writing Through Reading*,
Prentice-Hall, a developmental reading and
composition text.

1985 (with Cecile Forte) *Discovering Process*, Macmillan,
a composition rhetoric, integrating reading.

1990 (with Lowell Kleiman) *Philosophy: An Introduction
Through Literature*. Paragon House. An introductory
philosophy text, still being used at a number of
colleges and universities.

2014 *Templates*, Broadview Press, a sentence level
rhetoric.

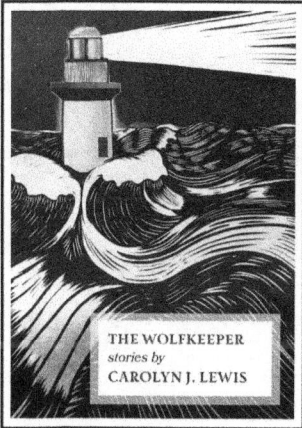

The Wolfkeeper: stories in this collection were nominated for the Pushcart Prize and were semi-finalists in Pirate's Alley William Faulkner awards and the Heekin Group Foundation's Tara Fellowship in Short Fiction.